# Paediatric Radiography

Maryann Hardy
*MSc, BSc(Hons), DCR*

Stephen Boynes
*MSc, BSc(Hons), TDCR*

*School of Health Studies, University of Bradford, UK*

**Blackwell**
Science

© 2003 by Blackwell Science Ltd
a Blackwell Publishing company

Editorial offices:
Blackwell Science Ltd,
9600 Garsington Road,
Oxford OX4 2DQ, UK
    Tel: +44 (0)1865 776868
Blackwell Publishing Inc.,
350 Main Street, Malden,
MA 02148-5020, USA
    Tel: +1 781 388 8250
Blackwell Science Asia Pty,
550 Swanston Street, Charlton,
Victoria 3053, Australia
    Tel: +61 (0)3 8359 1011

First published 2003

Library of Congress
Cataloging-in-Publication Data
Hardy, Maryann.
    Paediatric radiography/Maryann Hardy,
    Stephen Boynes.
    p.   cm.
    Includes bibliographical references and index.
    ISBN 0-632-05631-2 (hbk.)
    1.  Pediatric radiography.    2.  Diagnostic
    imaging.   3.  Pediatrics.   I.  Title: Pediatric
    radiography.   II.  Boynes, Stephen.   III.  Title.

    RJ51.R3 .H37 2003
    618.92′07572-dc21
                                        2002038606

ISBN 0-632-05631-2

A catalogue record for this title is available
from the British Library

Set in 10/12.5 Palatino
by SNP Best-set Typesetter Ltd, Hong Kong
Printed and bound in Great Britain by
Butler & Tanner Ltd, Frome and London

For further information on
Blackwell Publishing, visit our website:
www.blackwellpublishing.com

# Contents

# Preface

Paediatric radiography, despite being acknowledged as an imaging specialism, does not have a strong presence in either undergraduate or postgraduate radiography education programmes, and the availability of current published literature aimed at general radiographers is extremely limited. Consequently, the aim of *Paediatric Radiography* is to provide a reference text for radiographers and student radiographers working within general imaging departments and highlights aspects of paediatric healthcare that may influence paediatric radiography practice.

Importantly, when writing this text, we have not sought to provide a description of all paediatric imaging techniques or provide answers to all imaging dilemmas, because many of these will be dependent upon local expertise, radiographic equipment and availability of alternative imaging modalities. Instead we have attempted to raise important aspects of paediatric healthcare that should inform radiographic practice and hope that these will be discussed openly within imaging departments. As a consequence of the current shortage of paediatric radiography texts we have considered literature from other health professions, particularly nursing, and have attempted to adopt some of their good practice models. Therefore this text may also be useful for nurses, physiotherapists and junior doctors interested in the imaging of children and its role in current paediatric healthcare practice.

The development of this book has enriched our understanding of paediatric healthcare and the role of diagnostic imaging within the discipline. Our hope is that this book will help enhance paediatric radiographic practice to ensure that children attending imaging departments will receive informed and appropriate paediatric care.

*Maryann Hardy and Stephen Boynes*

# Acknowledgements

We are particularly grateful to Jonathan McConnell of St Martin's College, Lancaster and Anne-Marie Dixon of the University of Bradford for willingly sharing their knowledge of trauma and abdominal ultrasound respectively. In addition, we would like to thank Sue Watson, Andy Scally and Gary Culpan for critically reading appropriate chapters and providing comments and suggestions.

Special thanks are also due to Dr Rosemary Arthur, paediatric consultant radiologist at the General Infirmary at Leeds for providing information and images for inclusion within the text, and Dr Leanne Elliott, consultant radiologist at Bradford Royal Infirmary, who willingly gave us regular access to the paediatric film library housed within her office!

We would also like to offer our thanks to Gill Marles, Superintendent Radiographer, Clarendon Wing X-ray Department, the General Infirmary at Leeds, for allowing us access to the department for photographic purposes, and also to those patients and their families who consented to being photographed. In addition, thanks must go to the young models who were patient with us during very long photographic sessions; Benjamin Hardy, Peter Hardy, Robin Errington, Eve Errington, Alexander Errington, Benjamin Lodge, Jody Lodge and Theo Scally.

Thanks are also due to the staff of the following imaging departments who allowed us to watch them work and were open in discussions around techniques:

> Clarendon Wing X-ray Department, The General Infirmary at Leeds
> Sheffield Children's Hospital
> Manchester Children's Hospital (Booth Hall)
> Hull A&E Department
> Bradford Royal Infirmary

# Chapter 1
# Understanding childhood

A child is, as defined by English law, any person under the age of 18 years. It is assumed that by the age of 18 a person has reached such a level of maturity as to be capable of making fully informed decisions. However, it is the process of growth and development during childhood and adolescence that results in maturity and not chronological age alone.

Growth is the progressive development of a living being, or any part of it, from its earliest stage to maturity[1]. In health care we usually restrict the term to mean the physiological and anatomical changes that occur. Growth is not constant. Different parts of the human body grow at different rates and the growth of one system can be affected by the activity of another (e.g. human growth hormone produced by the endocrine system affects growth within the musculoskeletal system). In contrast, the term development is commonly used to describe the psychological and cognitive advancement of a child and the acquisition of motor and sensory skills.

Growth and development are variables of childhood and children of the same age can be at different growth and developmental stages. Consequently, when deciding the most appropriate health care approach it is important to allow for a child's individuality and to avoid making assumptions about a child based upon preconceived ideas pertaining to specific chronological ages. However, although children of the same age can be at different developmental stages, the order in which growth and development occurs is generally consistent for all children[2]. For example, ossification of the carpus occurs in the same order for all children, but the exact age at which the carpal bones ossify can vary markedly.

As a result of predictable developmental staging, many texts, including this one, have provided general growth and development charts that are loosely linked to chronological age. Figures 1.1 and 1.2 have been designed to highlight important stages in growth and development that may be useful to clinical radiographers and to indicate the approximate ages at which they occur. These charts are not definitive and radiographers should not rely upon them solely but should combine them with a general understanding of the child development process. The inclusion of school children and adolescents in Fig. 1.2 has been purposeful as although radiographic technique may not vary dramatically from that used for adults, the radiographer's approach to the patient will need to be modified. Appreciating the social, physical and cognitive developments that occur during these phases of childhood will assist the radiographer in selecting a suitable approach to the examination and will ensure appropriate and effective patient communication and co-operation.

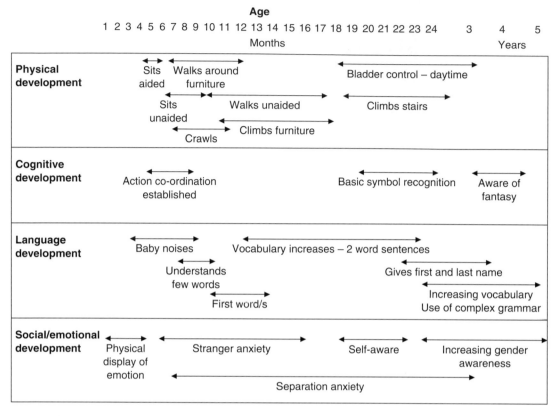

**Fig. 1.1**  Growth and development staging chart (birth–5 years).

# Physical growth

The peculiarity of growth is what physically differentiates a child from an adult. Infants grow rapidly in the first year of life, increasing their body length by approximately 50%. Between 1 and 2 years of age, a child's height increases by approximately 12 cm and thereafter, until puberty, children increase in height by approximately 6 cm per annum. The onset of puberty is associated with a sudden and marked increase in growth (the adolescence spurt) and this phase lasts for approximately 2 to 3 years in both boys and girls.

It is not only height that varies with age but also body proportion. Each organ or system grows at a different rate and therefore the relationship between one part of a growing body and another changes over time[3]. These changing body proportions are evident in Fig. 1.3. It is important to note that at birth the head and upper body are larger and functionally more advanced than the lower body. As the child grows, a leaner shape with longer legs is gradually adopted and the relative size of the upper body and head decreases.

The rate at which growth occurs varies between children and is also inconsistent within an individual child. Growth is episodic rather than constant and

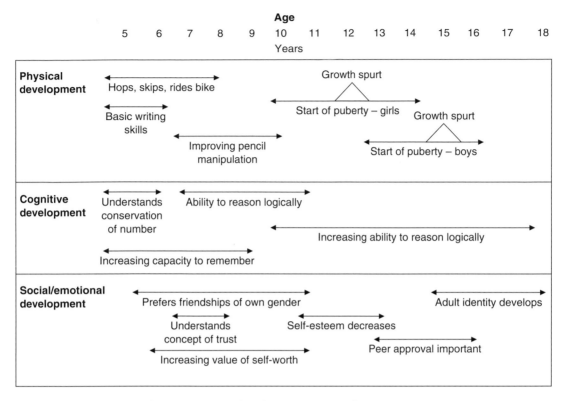

**Fig. 1.2** Growth and development staging chart (5 years–18 years).

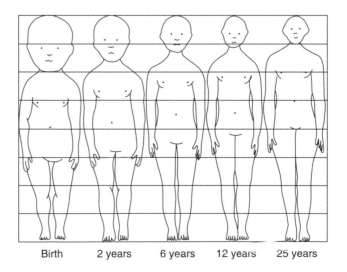

**Fig. 1.3** Changes in body proportions from birth to adulthood.

therefore results in growth spurts. The natural cyclic nature of growth can be adversely affected by serious childhood illness, resulting in decreased growth, and in some children noticeable growth retardation, but upon recovery these children will usually experience a period of accelerated growth until their 'normal' height has been achieved. The causes and reasons for episodic rather than constant growth are not yet understood and research in this area continues. However, it appears that each child carries an internal 'blue print' that determines their correct growth/height at a particular age and this is likely to be linked to hereditary and environmental factors.

# Psychological and cognitive development

A variety of child development theories have been proposed but, since the 1960s, education theory of child development in the UK has been dominated by Piaget's cognitive development theory. Piaget believed that the development of cognitive ability (acquisition of knowledge including perception, intuition and reasoning) occurred in sequential stages and he linked these to the chronological age of a child rather than to the intellectual or emotional maturity of the child as favoured by modern theorists.

Cognitive development, like physical growth, is individual to the child and their personal experiences. However, a child's level of cognition directly influences their understanding of, and reaction to, illness[4] and there is considerable evidence that a child's interpretation of health and illness progresses systematically[5]. However, because not all children have the same experiences, some children will understand more than others at each age. As a result, age is not a good, nor an accurate, indicator of understanding.

## Birth to 3 years

A very young child has little direct understanding of illness but during this period strong attachments to family members are made and children experience stranger and separation anxiety when in new and unfamiliar situations. To maintain the security and comfort of the child it is important to include the guardians in the care of their child. Explanation of the procedure should be made in a friendly manner and facial expressions should be welcoming. The attention span and memory of a toddler is short and therefore distraction techniques (e.g. bubbles and pop-up books) may need to be considered as a tool to ensure a high-quality examination (see Chapter 2).

## 3 to 7 years

Children within this age group perceive illness to be an external occurrence but different levels of perception exist and understanding is enhanced by education and experience of illness. Explanation of a procedure should be made using language that the child will understand and the use of pictures, books and toys to aid explanation[5] and a demonstration of equipment to be used (if possible) will help allay fears and gain the child's co-operation[6]. Children in this age group will still require the support of a guardian in strange situations and this involvement should be encouraged.

## 7 to 11 years

The ability to understand and reason improves within this age range and any display of lack of understanding may have more to do with a lack of specific knowledge than immature development[7]. Care needs to be taken not to undermine the child and to provide appropriate information that will allow comprehension and understanding of the medical procedure. For these children, fear of the unknown is still a real problem but expression of this fear or other emotion may be difficult and so a display of 'bravado' may occur to mask inner uncertainties. It is important for radiographers to appreciate that children may 'put on an act' of confidence when in strange situations but they will still require considerable care and attention and the involvement and support of a guardian.

## Adolescents

The young adolescent experiences many emotional and physical changes and early adolescence is often associated with a period of low self-esteem and self-doubt[8]. These young people are much more sensitive and socially self-conscious than any other age group and therefore have particular needs within the health care setting. A major cause of this sensitivity is the onset of puberty.

During the pubescent stage, the young adolescent is egocentric and physically self-conscious, not wanting to be perceived as different from his or her peers. Confidentiality and privacy is particularly important and reassurance and support is required from the health care professional[9]. Many young adolescents will want to have their guardian present during examination, particularly if it is an invasive procedure, but, as they progress through adolescence, they may prefer to be accompanied by a health care chaperone of the same sex. It should not be assumed that the teenager will or will not wish to be accompanied by a guardian and the choice, where possible, should be offered to the adolescent.

Middle adolescents (15–17 years) are more confident of their personal identity, although those who, through disease or illness, are perceived to be 'different from the norm' will still require substantial emotional support. During this phase, a subculture of experimentation and boundary testing exists[10]. A consistent approach to the examination and a non-judgemental attitude is required of the radiographer dealing with this age group. The teenager should be involved in any decision-making process regarding their health care treatment and indeed, in English law, young people of age 16 years or older have the right to consent to medical, surgical and dental treatment (see Chapter 2). The end of this phase results in transition to late adolescence/adulthood and this stage brings with it new responsibilities and challenges (e.g. first job, learning to drive, sexual relationships). Unfortunately, it is also the stage at which the frequency of psycho-social disorders (e.g. depression) increases[11] and therefore radiographers need to be sensitive to the continuing emotional needs of the young patient.

# Role of family

The health of a child is dependent not only on the child's physical and mental well-being, but is also influenced by cultural, social and environmental factors. In the past patients, including children, have been treated as clinical cases rather than individuals in their own right, and attention has been given almost exclusively to the medical condition. The emphasis within health care has now changed and children are treated not only as individuals but also as part of a family, community and culture. This change has not occurred overnight but has resulted from a number of initiatives to involve guardians and family in the care of hospitalised children and to help the family maintain normal functioning (family centred care)[12].

The Department of Health document *Welfare of Children and Young People in Hospital*[13] and the Audit Commission document *Children First: A Study of Hospital Services*[14] both promote family centred care as the essential ethos behind successful paediatric nursing. Unfortunately, the term 'family centred care', although commonly used within the literature, has yet to be successfully defined. However, the ethos of family centred care (involving and caring for the whole family) underpins current paediatric nursing theory and aims to facilitate care based upon the needs of the child *and* his/her family[15]. Its implementation has been successful for families with hospitalised children, and guardians are becoming more actively involved in the nursing care and treatment of their child. However, within the acute setting its success has been limited and it has been suggested that alternative approaches to family centred care need to be devised if successful partnerships between guardians and health professionals are to be achieved[16]. Radiographers, therefore, need to consider their working practices and introduce new ways of including guardians in the examination process if successful short-term partnerships are to be achieved.

Accepting this partnership in the care of child patients has not been easy for paediatric health professionals and, in particular, the changes that have occurred within nursing, from primarily undertaking all clinical care tasks to negotiating and agreeing care plans with guardians, have developed over a period of years. Family centred care empowers the guardians and involves them in the care and health decisions pertaining to their child[17]. The philosophy for this is that it is in the child's best interests to be cared for by their family as this facilitates and promotes the continuation of normal family function. Unfortunately, the reality of modern lifestyles may prevent effective family care of a hospitalised child occurring (e.g. if the child is from a single parent family with other siblings at home then it may not be possible for the parent to be fully involved with the hospital care of the child) and it is important not to make guardians feel pressured or guilty if they are unable to fulfil the hospital carer role.

## Role of play

Play is an inherent part of childhood and a child's approach to play changes greatly in line with their physical and cognitive development, most particularly during preschool years[15]. Play is a part of the socialisation process allowing the child to imitate and experiment in the learning of social roles and values[7]. Unfortunately, a child's ability to play can be affected by illness, and immobility can leave a child frustrated, particularly in the generally active 7–11-year age group. To counteract this, professional play specialists are increasingly being employed to provide children with play opportunities suitable for their age and ability.

The role of the play specialist is now seen as essential to the care and well-being of hospitalised children and their role within the multidisciplinary team is increasingly being recognised. For example, they can take time to explain and demonstrate procedures to children (e.g. catheterisation procedure for a micturating cystogram can be demonstrated on a doll), time that often radiographers cannot spare, and they can suggest many easy ideas for distracting and comforting children during an examination. Their ability to incorporate play successfully into the daily care of hospitalised children has been shown to reduce anxiety and promote normality within an alien environment. Play has also been proven to be an invaluable tool in helping children understand procedures and treatments and enables both children and guardians to gain familiarity with unusual hospital equipment[18].

Unfortunately, play specialists are rarely found in radiology departments. Play equipment (books and toys) is commonly provided in waiting rooms but the standard and range of equipment varies and provision may only be made for the very youngest of children. It is essential that waiting areas are attractive and child-friendly environments. There should be opportunities for play appropriate to all ages[19] and particular attention should be paid to adolescents with regard to reading material. Whatever the play equipment provided within the department, it is essential that it is regularly inspected to ensure that broken toys and torn books are removed before they become hazardous to the child. It is also a psychological barrier to effective communication if the waiting room is untidy and available toys are broken or dirty. It is important that radiographers appreciate their working environment from the patient's viewpoint – in this case the child and guardian[5]. By sitting for a period of time in a waiting area or imaging room and looking at the environment with critical eyes it may be possible for simple, cheap improvements to be identified that will provide comfort to children of all ages without causing concern to other more mature patients.

## Summary

In summary, this chapter has aimed to outline some important features of growth and development in children in order to assist the radiographer in understanding the fears and anxiety of the young patient. It has also been important to introduce the concept of family centred care and emphasise the role of the family in the physical care and emotional support of a child as being of paramount importance in the modern National Health Service (NHS).

## References

1.  Sinclair, D. and Dangerfield, P. (1998) *Human Growth After Birth*, 6th edn. Oxford University Press, Oxford.
2.  Schickedanz, J.A. Schickedanz, D.I., Hansen, K. and Forsyth, P.D. (1993) *Understanding Children: Infancy Through Pre-School*, 2nd edn. Mayfield Publishing Company, London.
3.  Behram, R.E. and Kliegman, R.M. (1998) *Essentials of Pediatrics*, 3rd edn. WB Saunders Company, London.
4.  Swanwick, M. (1990) Knowledge and control. *Paediatric Nursing* **2** (5), 18–20.
5.  Taylor, J. and Muller, D.J. (1999) *Nursing Children: Psychology, Research and Practice*, 3rd edn. Stanley Thornes (Publishers) Ltd, Cheltenham.
6.  Carter, B. (1994) *Child and Infant Pain: Principles of Nursing Care and Management.* Chapman & Hall, London.
7.  Carter, B. and Dearmun, A.K. (eds) (1995) *Child Health Care Nursing: Concepts, Theory & Practice.* Blackwell Science, Oxford.
8.  Bee, H. (1999) *The Growing Child*, 2nd edn. Longman, Harlow.
9.  Marks, M.G. (1998) *Broadribb's Introductory Pediatric Nursing*, 5th edn. Lippincott, New York.
10. McQuade, L., Huband, S. and Parker, E. (1996) *Children's Nursing.* Churchill Livingstone, London.
11. Department of Health (1996) *Focus on Teenagers: Research Into Practice.* HMSO, Norwich.
12. Casey, A. (1988) A partnership with child and family. *Senior Nurse* **8** (4), 8–9.
13. Department of Health (1991) *Welfare of Children and Young People in Hospital.* HMSO, London.
14. Audit Commission (1993) *Children First: A Study of Hospital Services.* HMSO, London.
15. Bee, H. (2000) *The Developing Child*, 9th edn. Allyn and Bacon, London.
16. Coyne, I.T. (1996) Parent participation: a concept analysis. *Journal of Advanced Nursing* **23**, 733–40.
17. Hutchfield, K. (1999) Family-centred care: a concept analysis. *Journal of Advanced Nursing* **29** (5), 1178–87.
18. Cook, P. (1999) *Supporting Sick Children and Their Families.* Baillière Tindall, London.
19. Hogg, C. (1996) *Health Services for Children and Young People: A Guide for Commissioners and Providers*, Vol. 1. Action for Sick Children, Edinburgh.

# Chapter 2
# Consent, immobilisation and health care law

As health care professionals, radiographers have a duty of care towards patients whom they examine and UK government directives have emphasised the need for high-quality care and service for all patients[1,2]. The perception of quality is subjective and dependent upon the individual needs of the patient, therefore it is essential that radiographers work together with patients towards achieving a level of appropriate care. The ethos of family centred care currently underpins and drives high-quality patient care within dedicated paediatric units (see Chapter 1) but the application of this principle within the acute setting is not without difficulties. However, it is the responsibility of every health care practitioner (including radiographers) to ensure that the standard of care delivered is of high quality and is appropriate to the age and level of understanding displayed by the paediatric patient. This chapter aims to consider the legal aspects of health care, with particular regard to children's rights and immobilisation, and will consider distraction and alternative holding techniques as a method of reducing the need for forced immobilisation of the young child and ultimately improving the quality of patient care.

## Children's rights

Perceptions of children's rights are not universally consistent and it was the goal of the United Nations Convention on the Rights of the Child 1989 to clarify children's rights. Three important articles for health care workers within this convention are identified in Box 2.1.

**Box 2.1** From the United Nations Convention on the Rights of the Child[3].

*Article 3*: In all actions concerning children, the best interests of the child shall be a primary consideration.

*Article 12*: Parties shall assure to the child who is capable of forming his/her own views the right to express those views freely in all matters affecting the child, the views of the child being given due weight in accordance with age and maturity of the child.

*Article 24*: Parties shall take all effective and appropriate measures with a view to abolishing traditional practices prejudicial to the health of children.

The UK government, although ratifying the United Nations Convention on the Rights of the Child in 1991, has not yet fully embraced the rights of children to be involved in the decision-making process (article 12). The fundamental ideology of UK government policy is that of the protectionist, assuming that children need protecting from themselves[4]. The result of this is a belief that children are usually incapable of exercising choice and that children's rights should be invested in those with parental responsibility[5]. However, current interpretations of health care law do not fully support this view and recent government publications have acknowledged that patients have a right to be involved in the medical decision-making process (Kennedy Report, 2001) although it is unclear how and if this will affect the child patient. As a consequence, radiographers need to be aware of, and appreciate, both the concepts of patients' rights and children's rights within the health care setting and their current (and future) incorporation into health care law.

# Health care law

Under UK law, every competent adult has a right to give or to refuse consent to medical treatment and, in the absence of consent, the fact that an action was taken in the 'best interests of the patient' would not be a valid defence[6]. UK law also allows an adult to make an 'irrational' decision (that is one that would not accord with the decision of the vast majority of people), without this leading to the conclusion that the person lacks the capacity to make a valid choice[7].

Regarding children, UK law is more complicated. The Family Law Reform Act 1969, section 8, gives 16 and 17 year-olds the right to consent to medical, dental and surgical treatment. Such consent cannot be overridden by those with parental responsibility for the child. For children under 16 years of age, no provision to consent to medical treatment was given in law until 1985 when the UK law lords determined that a 'Gillick competent' child did have the capacity to consent to medical treatment (*Gillick* v. *W. Norfolk AHA*).

'Gillick competence' is achieved when a child is deemed to have sufficient understanding and intelligence to enable him or her to fully understand the treatment being proposed. It requires an appreciation of the consequences of treatment, including side effects and anticipated consequences of a failure to treat[8], but it does *not* introduce the need for moral maturity. The test for 'understanding' is not whether a wise decision would be made but whether the child is capable of making a choice[9].

Despite the term 'test', there is no objective tool to measure a child's competence. In most circumstances, it is the responsibility of the health care professional to make a judgement[10] based upon subjective personal opinions and there lies the fundamental flaw. It has been suggested that, rather than try to prove competence, we should assume competence and attempt to disprove it[11] and in 1996, Alderson and Montgomery proposed the adoption of a Children's Code of Practice for Healthcare Right's which assumed children of compulsory school age were competent, therefore placing responsibility on the health care professional to justify 'ignoring' the views of the child[12]. So far this code has not been approved.

'Gillick competence' is of fundamental importance within the 1989 Children Act which aimed to clarify children's health and social legal issues. The Children Act laid down that *'children who are judged able to give consent* can not *be medically examined and treated without their consent'*[13]. The implication of this was that competent children could refuse to be medically examined or treated.

Since the introduction of the Children Act, the issue of consent by the competent child has arisen on numerous occasions and with it have been considerations of the rights and responsibilities of the parents of a 'Gillick competent' child. Lord Scarman stated that 'the parental right to determine whether or not their minor below the age of 16 will have medical treatment terminates if and when the child achieves a sufficient understanding and intelligence to fully understand what is being proposed'. Lord Donaldson challenged this interpretation and suggested that there was still the power for parents to approve treatment in the face of the child's refusal and he asserted his view that 'parents do not lose the power to consent when children become competent'[9].

Lord Donaldson's statement that parental rights to consent persist after a child has become competent becomes important in the situation where a child refuses medical treatment. In such circumstances, even in the 16 and 17 years age group, a person with parental responsibility can consent to treatment on behalf of a child who is refusing treatment. Such parental authorisation will enable the treatment to be undertaken but will not *require* the practitioner to do so[14], as in all circumstances the practitioner must act in what they believe are the best interests of the child.

Health care law is very confusing and much work needs to be undertaken to ensure it is 'fit for purpose'. Essentially, children under 16 years of age do not have the right to consent or refuse treatment unless they have achieved Gillick competence, a test for which does not exist, and the assessment of which is in the hands of the health care professional who may or may not have paediatric experience. Children of ages 16 and 17 years can, in law, consent to medical treatment whether or not they are competent. No child of any age can refuse medical treatment that has been consented to by a person with parental responsibility and this ruling can also be applied to diagnostic procedures that are necessary to determine what treatment, if any, is necessary. However, parental consent does not necessarily mean that a child will permit examination and therefore, as a last resort, it may be necessary to consider immobilisation of the child in order to facilitate appropriate examination or treatment.

## Immobilisation versus restraint

The term 'restraint' is generally reserved for use within the mental health setting. The more general terminology used within health care is 'immobilisation'.

To immobilise a person is to render them fixed or incapable of moving[15] whereas restraint is the forcible confinement[16], limitation or restriction[17]. From these definitions, it is clear that the difference between the two terms is the degree of force necessary to accomplish the restriction. Therefore it may be useful to determine immobilisation as that restriction to which the child has consented by permitting contact, and restraint as forced restriction to which the child has not consented (even though parental consent may have been received). With this understanding, it is possible to speculate that although the term immobilisation is used within the general health care setting, paediatric restraint could be occasionally undertaken in order to achieve diagnostic radiographic images, and although not politically correct, this would concur with the views of European guidelines[18].

During the 1990s, European research identified that the most frequent causes of inadequate and poor-quality imaging of children were incorrect radiographic positioning and unsuccessful immobilisation of paediatric patients[19]. As a result of this research, European Guidelines on Quality Criteria for Diagnostic Radiographic Images in Paediatrics were issued[18]. These guidelines state that patient positioning, prior to exposure to radiation, must be exact whether or not the patient co-operates. The guidelines advocate the use of physical restraints in the immobilisation of young children and state that for infants, toddlers and young children, immobilisation devices, properly applied, must ensure that the patient does not move and the correct projection is achieved. However, experience within UK imaging departments has shown that immobilisation devices that rely on the child being strapped into position are rarely efficient in achieving adequate immobilisation in children over 3 months of age[20] without the co-operation of the child and guardian[21].

The restraint and immobilisation of children raises many ethical and professional considerations. Restraint compromises the dignity and liberty of the child and therefore to restrain a child solely to facilitate examination, rather than concern that the child may cause serious bodily harm to himself/herself or another, may not be ethical[22]. In 1996, Robinson and Collier[23] researched the educational and ethical issues perceived by nurses with regard to 'holding patients still' and found that nurses did have concerns in this regard, particularly as the majority felt it was the restraint and not pain that caused the most distress to the child. Nurses were also unclear of their legal position with respect to restraining children for medical procedures. As a result of this research, the Royal College of Nurses issued guidelines entitled *Restraining, Holding Still and Containing Children. Guidance for Good Practice*[24]. Although these guidelines clearly differentiate 'holding still' from restraint, they do not clarify the legal position of health care professionals involved in the holding of paediatric patients, nor do they provide practical advice on appropriate holding techniques to be employed when working with children.

## Holding children still – a five-point model

Little research has been published that evaluates techniques in holding and comforting children, even though it is generally agreed that all health professionals working with children need education and training into the immobilisation and

**Box 2.2**   A five-point model of child comfort and immobilisation.

| |
|---|
| (1)   Prepare child and guardian for procedure and explain their role |
| (2)   Invite guardian to be present |
| (3)   Use a specific room for painful procedures |
| (4)   Position child in a comforting manner |
| (5)   Maintain a calm and positive atmosphere |

distraction of children[25]. To this end, Stephens *et al.*[26] designed a five-point model of child comfort and immobilisation for nursing procedures which can be adapted to meet the needs of other health disciplines (Box 2.2).

### Prepare child and guardian

Attending for a medical examination within a hospital environment is a major event in the lives of most children and therefore radiographers should approach the child in a serious but friendly manner, understanding that the role of the radiographer is not to make the child happy but to offer reassurance, inspire confidence and provide appropriate information.

Before the radiographic examination commences, both the child and guardian need to know why the examination is necessary, what the procedure will be and essentially what their role will be (i.e. what is expected of them). It is often difficult for radiographers with limited experience of children to provide explanations at a level appropriate to the child and this difficulty is compounded by the fact that in stressful situations children will often regress to a younger developmental age. It is not, therefore, appropriate to use chronological age alone as a guide to the level of explanation but instead an assessment of the apparent developmental age displayed by the child needs to be made.

Taking time to explain the procedure is essential if maximum co-operation is to be achieved and the use of physical restraints minimised. The explanation should, if possible, be made in a neutral environment such as the waiting area and, as the age at which comprehension begins is uncertain, it should be worded in such a way as to be understandable to both adult and child, including children as young as 12 months of age (Fig. 2.1).

An effective explanation, although apparently time consuming, will in fact result in a more efficient examination as improved child and guardian co-operation will reduce actual examination time and, if the explanation can be undertaken outside of the imaging room, will reduce patient waiting times. A possible approach to effective explanation is given in Box 2.3.

### Invite guardian to be present

Family centred care (see Chapter 1) is the major ethos of children's healthcare today and working in partnership with guardians is seen as essential if high-quality care is to be provided and maintained. The presence of a guardian within

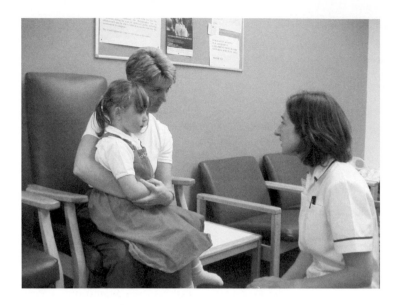

**Fig. 2.1** The radiographer is positioned at the level of the child in order to engage the child and effectively explain the procedure to both child and guardian.

**Box 2.3**  An approach to effective explanation.

- Remove distractions
- Sit facing the child and guardian and speak in a quiet voice with a serious tone
- Behave as if this examination is of maximum importance
- Explain the procedure to guardian and child and define their roles (i.e. what you want them to do). A guardian will be able to comfort and divert a child more effectively if they understand what is happening
- Emphasise the child's role is to remain still throughout the examination and repeat this role at several intervals during the explanation
- Provide the child with choices to emphasise their control of the situation (e.g. 'Who do you want to come with you?', 'Do you want to bring your teddy?' or 'Do you want to sit on a chair or dad's knee?')

the examination room provides the child with security and it has been found that 99% of 5–12 year-olds believe that the presence of their guardian will help reduce pain and anxiety[27]. Guardians are also able to comfort the child in a familiar manner and often instinctively implement appropriate distraction techniques that can reduce the child's fear and anxiety, increase the child's co-operation and minimise the need for restraining devices.

*Position child in a comforting manner*

Lying supine within an unfamiliar environment increases the feeling of helplessness and loss of control in adults and children alike and increases patient anxiety. Radiographers need to be more creative in their imaging strategies when examining children and work with what is presented rather than 'forcing' the child to adopt a position routinely used in the imaging of adults. The need for 'cuddles' and comfort throughout an imaging examination is not restricted to very young children and children as old as 7 or 8 years will prefer to sit across a guardian's lap or next to a guardian to gain comfort from their presence (Figs 2.2–2.5).

## Maintain a calm, positive atmosphere

If you talk to a screaming child quietly and positively then eventually they will calm down. Anxiety levels in children and adults increase with the level of surrounding noise and therefore focusing on a calm and quiet voice can help reduce this anxiety.

## Distraction tools

The use of distraction techniques within health care is growing greater in prominence and the experts in the use of distraction and play are play specialists. Play specialists are not generally employed within imaging departments but instead tend to work mainly on children's wards and outpatient clinics. However, most play specialists would welcome the opportunity to discuss child-friendly environments and distraction techniques with other health care professionals and

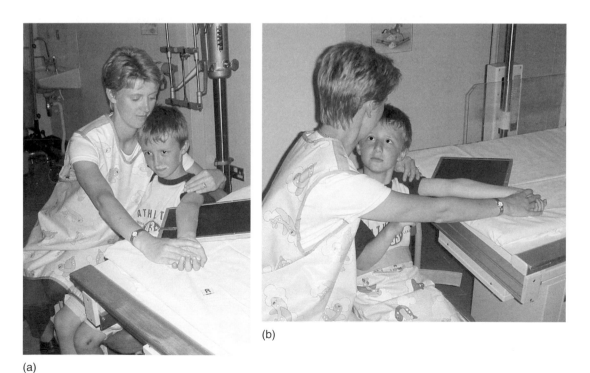

(a)

(b)

**Fig. 2.2**   (a) and (b) Sitting an older child next to the guardian allows them to feel comforted while still respecting their 'older' status. The guardian can also assist with immobilisation.

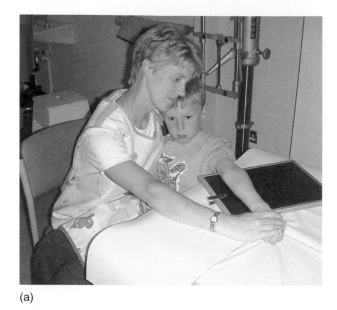

(a)

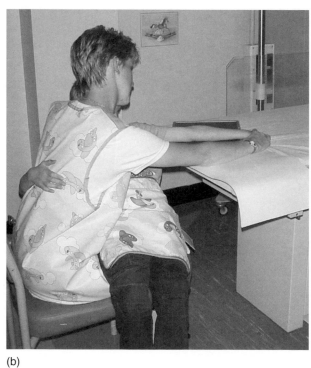

(b)

**Fig. 2.3** (a) and (b) Sitting the child across the guardian's lap is a natural and comforting position for older children and permits some adult assistance with positioning and immobilisation. Note the guardian and child are seated to the side of the table.

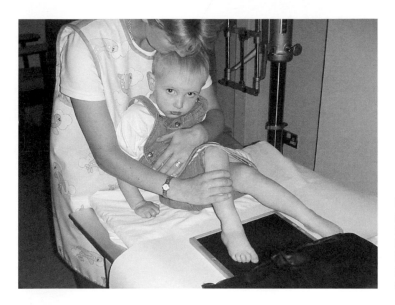

**Fig. 2.4** Seating a young child at the end of the table where they can 'lean in' to the guardian is more comforting than being laid in the supine position and may be useful for examinations of the lower limb.

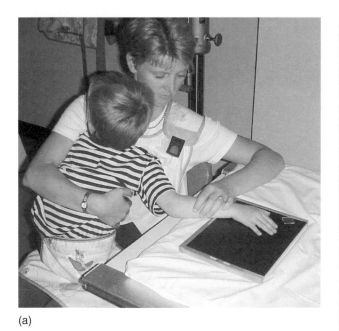

(a)

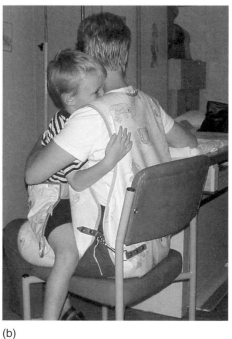

(b)

**Fig. 2.5** (a) and (b) The straddle hold is a natural, comforting position for young children and naturally allows the guardian to successfully immobilise the child and assist in positioning.

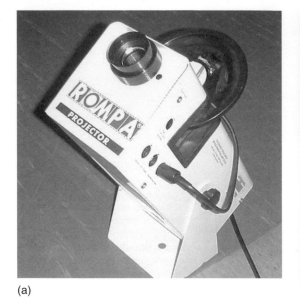

(a)

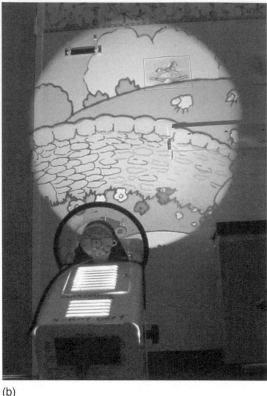

(b)

**Fig. 2.6**   (a) and (b) Projectors may be useful distraction tools within the x-ray room but care needs to be taken to ensure that they are positioned in a safe and appropriate place without electrical leads trailing across the room.

should be contacted to advise on the needs of children within radiology depart-ments. Alternatively, various pieces of equipment designed to distract children are available but care must be taken before purchase to ensure that they are easy to use and operate (Fig. 2.6). Whatever the distraction tools used, it is essential that they be used only within the examination room to maintain their novelty value and maximise their effectiveness.

Whatever their age, children have a right to receive care that offers the most comfort available, whether that comfort be physical or psychological. It is also important that radiographers appreciate that adolescents are not adults and can, during times of severe stress or trauma, regress to a much younger age.

## Summary

Children's rights within health care are confused and limited. In reality, children only have the right to agree to a treatment and, for those under 16 years of age, this is only if they have met some subjective measure of competence. Although the 1989 Children Act made steps to advance children's rights, subsequent law lord rulings have in essence reversed the direction of children's rights to a point where, with respect to the refusal of medical examination, the Children Act is contradicted.

Immobilisation and restraint are not medical treatments in themselves and the ethics of restraining a child purely to facilitate treatment have been questioned in this chapter. It is possible that a competent child may consent to immobilisation but, if a child refuses to co-operate, it can be inferred from current law that, with parental consent, restraint is permissible in order to facilitate examination. However, restraint must only be applied if the treatment is *beyond doubt* in the best interests of the child.

It is essential that in the future, we involve children and their families in the decision-making process to ensure that a high-quality radiographic service is being delivered, and we can begin this process by working with families to ensure patient understanding and co-operation is achieved through effective communication and consideration of the child's need for comfort and support throughout the imaging examination.

# References

1. Department of Health (1997) *A First Class Service: Quality in the New NHS.* Department of Health, London.
2. Department of Health (2000) *The NHS Plan: A Plan For Investment, A Plan For Reform.* Department of Health, London.
3. United Nations (1989) *Convention on the Rights of the Child.* United Nations Publishing Office, Luxembourg.
4. Fulton, Y. (1996) Children's rights and the role of the nurse. *Paediatric Nursing* **8** (10), 29–31.
5. Payne, M. (1995) Children's rights and children's needs. *Health Visitor* **68** (10), 412–14.
6. Dimond, B. (1996) *The Legal Aspects of Child Health Care.* Mosby, London.
7. Rogers, W.V.H. (1994) *Winfield & Jolowicz on TORT*, 14th edn. Sweet & Maxwell, London.
8. Medical Defence Union (1997) *Consent to Treatment.* Medical Defence Union, London.
9. Montgomery, J. (1997) *Health Care Law.* Oxford University Press, Oxford.
10. College of Radiographers (1995) *The Implications for Radiographers of the Children Act.* College of Radiographers, London.
11. Alderson, P. (1993) *Children's Consent to Surgery.* Open University Press, Buckingham.
12. Alderson, P. and Montgomery, J. (1996) What about me? *Health Service Journal* 11/4/96, 22–4.
13. Department of Health (1990) *DoH circular HC(90)22* in *The Children Act 1989 – An Introductory Guide for the NHS.* HMSO, London.
14. Brazier, M. (1992) *Medicine, Patients and the Law.* Penguin Books, London.
15. *Stedman's Medical Dictionary* (1999, 26th edn). Williams & Wilkins, London.
16. *Dorland's Illustrated Medical Dictionary* (1988, 27th edn). WB Saunder's Company, London.
17. *The Collins Dictionary and Thesaurus* (1987) William Collins Sons & Co. Ltd, London.
18. Kohn, M.M., Moores, B.M., Schibilla, H. *et al.* (eds) (1996) *European Guidelines on*

*Quality Criteria for Diagnostic Radiographic Images in Paediatrics* (EUR 16261 EN). Office for Official Publications of the European Communities, Luxembourg.

19. Cook, J.V., Pettet, A., Shah, K. *et al.* (1998) *Guidelines on Best Practice in the X-ray Imaging of Children: A Manual For All X-ray Departments.* Queen Mary's Hospital for Children, The St Helier NHS Trust, Carshalton, Surrey and The Radiological Protection Centre, St George's Healthcare NHS Trust, London.

20. Gyll, C. and Blake, N. (1986) *Paediatric Diagnostic Imaging.* William Heinemann Medical Books, London.

21. Parkes, K. (1998) Paediatric trauma: dealing with young patients. *Synergy* (Oct), 6–7.

22. Harrison, C., Kenny, N.P., Sidarons, M. and Rowell, M. (1997) Bioethics for clinicians. 9: Involving children in medical decisions. *Canadian Medical Association Journal* **156**, 825–8.

23. Robinson, S. and Collier, J. (1997) Holding children still for procedures. *Paediatric Nursing* **9** (4), 12–14.

24. Royal College of Nurses (1999) *Restraining, Holding Still and Containing Children. Guidance for Good Practice.* Royal College of Nurses, London.

25. Collins, P. (1999) Restraining children for painful procedures. *Paediatric Nursing* **11** (3), 14–16.

26. Stephens, B.K., Barkey, M.E. and Hall, H.R. (1999) Techniques to comfort children during stressful procedures. *Accident & Emergency Nursing* **7**, 226–36.

27. Ross, D.M. and Ross, S.A. (1984) Childhood pain: the school-aged child's viewpoint. *Pain* **20**, 179–91.

# Chapter 3
# Radiation protection

Radiation protection in diagnostic radiography is essential if medical exposure to ionising radiation is to be maintained at a level of minimal acceptable risk[1]. The concept of risk is an important one and it is essential that we reduce risks to patient and staff through the justification, optimisation and limitation of radiation exposures (see Box 3.1)[2].

## Ionising radiation regulations

In the year 2000 the Ionising Radiation (Medical Exposure) Regulations (IR(ME))[3] were implemented in the UK. These regulations, together with the Ionising Radiations Regulations 1999[4] (IRR99), laid down basic measures to be implemented in order to protect individuals against the dangers of ionising radiations in relation to medical exposure.[3] The IR(ME) regulations specifically impose duties on those responsible for administering ionising radiation (e.g. radiographers) in order to protect persons undergoing a medical exposure whereas the IRR99 impose duties on employers to protect employees and other persons against occupational exposure to ionising radiation (some of these duties being by employment transferred to the employee)[4].

Together, these regulations, and more specifically regulations 32(1) and 32(3) of IRR99, make compulsory quality assurance programmes and radiation protection measures in order to minimise radiation exposure to staff, patients and guardians[3,4]. As part of this programme, national dose reference levels for diagnostic radiographic examinations are to be calculated thereby allowing local dose levels to be measured against nationally accepted dose levels and European norms. Through modification and improvement of techniques to ensure local doses are in line with those nationally recommended, this will standardise radiation exposure for specific radiographic examinations. However, it is likely that the national dose reference levels will, at least initially, be calculated only for the adult population as difficulties in establishing dose reference levels for paediatric examinations exist due to the wide variation in patient size and composition throughout the paediatric age range[5].

Even without national dose reference levels for paediatric examinations, there is much that can be done within clinical departments to ensure that unnecessary exposure to ionising radiation is minimised. The IR(ME) regulations emphasise the necessity for *justification and optimisation* of radiographic exposures as an essential step in the radiation protection process and stress that any examination that does not have a direct influence on patient management should not be undertaken. Unfortunately, unnecessary examinations are still requested by

**Box 3.1**   Definition of terms.

*Justification*:   No practice involving exposure to radiation should be adopted unless it produces net benefit to those exposed or to society

*Optimisation*:   Radiation doses and risks should be kept As Low As Reasonably Achievable (ALARA), economic and social factors being taken into account; constraints should be applied to dose or risk to prevent an unacceptable degree of exposure in any particular circumstance

*Limitation*:   The exposure of individuals should be subject to dose or risk limits above which the radiation risk would be deemed unacceptable

Adapted from National Radiation Protection Board (1994)[2]

clinicians who are unfamiliar with modern imaging techniques and concerns have been raised over the level of training in radiological techniques that currently exist within undergraduate medical courses[6].

Justification, as the first step in radiation protection, implies that the necessary diagnostic information cannot be obtained by other methods associated with a lower risk to the patient, and that there is sound clinical evidence to suggest that the patient will benefit from the investigation in terms of treatment and management[1]. It is important that any person justifying a radiation exposure has an understanding of the balance between the benefit and the risk of the exposure.

Once a diagnostic examination has been justified, the subsequent imaging process should be optimised by considering the interplay between three important aspects of the imaging process:

(1)   The diagnostic quality of the radiographic image
(2)   The radiation dose to the patient
(3)   The choice of radiographic technique

All three components need to be carefully considered if the quality and value of the imaging examination is to be optimised. However, differences in the anatomical and developmental features of a child, as well as varying body proportions, can make this task difficult and an understanding of the anatomical and developmental changes that occur during infancy, childhood and adolescence are essential. The European Guidelines on Quality Criteria for Diagnostic Radiographic Images in Paediatrics[5] presupposes that practising radiographers already have a knowledge of the changing radiographic anatomy of the developing child but much of this knowledge must be gained experientially as there are few texts to support learning in this area. As a result, radiographers who do not regularly examine children may have difficulty adapting radiographic anatomy from the adult patient to the child.

## Patient positioning

Incorrect positioning is the most frequent cause of inadequate radiographic image quality in paediatrics[5] and, although it is generally accepted that the correct positioning of paediatric patients can be much more difficult than positioning co-operative adult patients, this should not be used as an excuse for substandard image quality. The acceptability of an image as diagnostic depends upon the clinical question posed and it may be that, in certain circumstances, a lower level of image quality may be acceptable for certain clinical indications. However, inferior image quality cannot be justified unless it has been intentionally designed and is associated with a reduced radiation dose to the patient. The fact that the patient was unco-operative should not be used as an excuse for producing inferior quality images, which are often associated with excessive dose, as *no* diagnostic radiation exposure should be made unless there is a high probability that exact positioning has been achieved and will be maintained for the duration of the exposure (see Chapter 2).

## Field size and beam limitation

Inappropriate field size is a common fault in paediatric radiographic technique and correction is an effective method of reducing unnecessary dose to the patient. Correct beam limitation requires the radiographer to apply precise knowledge of external anatomical landmarks to the paediatric patient being examined. However, these landmarks vary with the physical growth and development of the child and are, therefore, not necessarily identical for children of similar ages. In addition, the field size depends much more on the nature of the underlying disease in infants and younger children than in adults (e.g. the lung fields may be extremely large in congestive heart failure and emphysematous pulmonary diseases whereas the diaphragm may be very high with intestinal meteorism, chronic obstruction or digestive diseases).

Accepting the importance of accurate collimation to the area of interest as a method of reducing dose is further emphasised in the European Guidelines on Quality Criteria for Diagnostic Radiographic Images in Paediatrics[5]. These guidelines state that the maximum field size tolerance should be less than 2 cm greater than the area of interest and this is further reduced to a tolerance of 1 cm in neonates. Consequently, appropriate quality assurance testing of mobile and stationary radiographic equipment to ensure that the light beam diaphragm correlates with the radiation beam is vital if consistent and accurate collimation is to be achieved.

## Protective shielding

For all paediatric examinations, the consistent use of lead rubber to shield that part of the body in immediate proximity to the diagnostic field is essential. Experimental data have shown that, when using exposures in the range of 60–80 kV, a reduction in gonadal dose of up to 40% can be achieved when 0.25 mm lead rubber equivalent is applied at the field edge[5]. However, this reduction in dose is only possible if the lead protection is placed at the field edge. Lead rubber covering placed further away is less effective and at a distance of 4 cm or more has been shown to be completely ineffective as a radiation protection measure[5].

For examinations where the gonads lie in or near (within 4 cm of) the primary radiation beam, lead protection should be applied whenever possible (Fig. 3.1). For boys, correctly positioned testicle capsules (Fig. 3.2) have been shown to

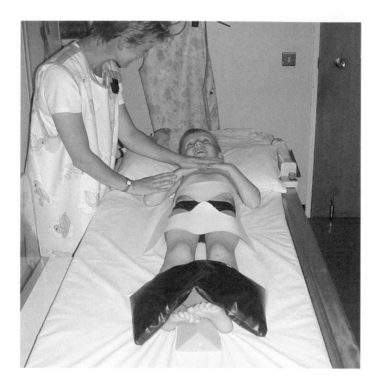

**Fig. 3.1**   Shaped lead protection used for radiography of the hips.

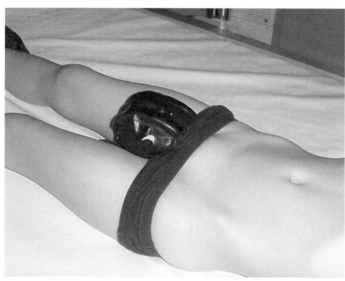

**Fig. 3.2**   Correct position of testicle capsule with effective use of underpant elastic to ensure testicles are below level of symphysis pubis.

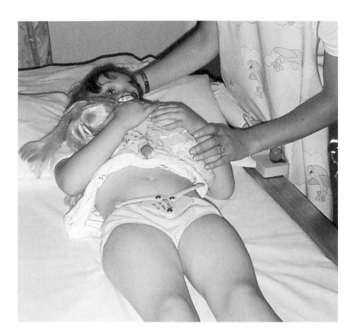

**Fig. 3.3**  Female gonad protection.
Note the child is cuddling a doll to aid
distraction, immobilisation and co-
operation.

reduce the testicular absorbed dose by up to 95%[5]. However, for this level of dose
reduction the testes must be secured within the scrotum, and if this is possible
then there is no reason to include the male gonads within the primary radiation
field for abdominal or pelvic radiographs. For girls, effective gonadal protection
is more difficult but correct positioning of lead protection shields can result in a
dose reduction to the ovaries of up to 50% (Fig. 3.3). However, it should be
remembered that the pelvis of a very young child is small and the bladder,
ovaries and uterus therefore lie just outside the pelvis.

Other anatomical regions that are particularly sensitive to radiation are the lens
of the eye and developing breast tissue. For radiography of the skull and face, the
postero-anterior projection can reduce the dose to the lens of the eyes by up to
95% and therefore postero-anterior skull techniques should be adopted as soon as
the patient's ability to co-operate permits. For radiography of the thorax and
spine effective dose reduction to the breast can also be achieved through postero-
anterior positioning of the patient and the traditional radiographic practice of
imaging the paediatric spine and chest antero-posterior should be questioned[5].

# Radiographic exposure parameters

## Focal spot size

If a choice of focal spot size is available, then the decision should be made upon
the ability of the focal spot to provide the most appropriate exposure time and
radiographic voltage selection at a stated focus-to-film distance (FFD) – this will
not always be the smaller focal spot.

### Tube filtration

Most x-ray tubes have installed as a minimum a 2.5 mm aluminium equivalent filtration. The effect of filtration is to absorb low-energy photons emitted from the anode, thereby reducing patient dose and increasing the quality of the beam. The use of a high kV technique is often desirable, but not all generators are capable of the short exposure times necessary. Where the range of selectable mA values is limited and where the minimum exposure time is 0.01 seconds or greater, it may be necessary to increase filtration to enable the selection of an appropriate higher kV without producing excessive film blackening.

It is recommended that the minimum additional filtration for paediatric examinations is 1 mm aluminium plus 0.1 mm copper[5], although this is dependent upon the filtration already incorporated within the tube and should be decided locally. This additional filtration need not be permanently placed within the x-ray tube but the facility made available to add filtration to the tube when required.

### Voltage

In spite of recommended high kV techniques, low kV paediatric examinations continue to be undertaken. High voltages facilitate the use of short exposure times and the extremely short exposure times needed for paediatric radiographic examinations can only be achieved if a high frequency (or 12-pulse) generator is used. The use of added filtration can allow the utilisation of high kV techniques with longer exposure times when operating older equipment (see 'Tube filtration' above).

### Anti-scatter grids

The use of anti-scatter grids in the radiographic examination of infants and young children is generally accepted as unnecessary. Paediatric examinations undertaken with the use of anti-scatter grids result in increased radiation dose to the patient and therefore their continued use should be questioned if diagnostic radiographs of satisfactory quality can be produced without them. Fluoroscopic equipment should also have the facility to quickly remove and insert grids and once again, the necessity of the use of a grid in the examination of young children should be questioned[7].

### Screen film systems

Although advancing technology is quickly bringing in the digital age, many imaging departments still operate a film/screen imaging system and therefore it is important to consider their value as a method of reducing patient dose. High-speed systems result in a lower patient dose and allow shorter exposure times to be used therefore minimising movement unsharpness. However, these obvious advantages must be balanced against the reduction in image resolution and detail that also occurs. The European Guidelines on Quality Criteria for Diagnostic Radiographic Images in Paediatrics[5] clearly advocate that film/screen systems with a speed class of less than 400 should not be used unless specific detail is necessary for accurate diagnosis. Cook *et al.* (1998) echo this view and they go further to state that where positional information only is required (e.g. the femoral head position in developmental dysplasia of the hip) then faster speed film/screen systems, which further reduce patient dose, can be used[7].

### Digital systems

Digital imaging technology permits a wide range of exposure parameters (and therefore patient doses) to be used without significantly affecting the perceived image quality. It is therefore essential that appropriate exposure parameters are established and adhered to in order to ensure minimum patient dose. Ideally the kV/mAs combination used should be sufficient to ensure that the noise in the image is just low enough for the image quality to be diagnostically acceptable.

### Automatic exposure control

Many automatic exposure control (AEC) systems commonly available are not suitable for paediatric imaging due to the large and relatively fixed position of the ionisation chambers. The constant growth that occurs during childhood results in changing body proportions and no fixed AEC device could be effectively used for all age ranges. Care also needs to be taken as many ionisation chambers are situated behind an anti-scatter grid and, if the grid is not removed prior to exposure, this will result in an increased patient dose. The use of exposure charts relating radiographic technique to patient weight (or age for extremity radiography) is likely to be a better option if dose reduction is to be successfully achieved.

### Automatic brightness control

Fluoroscopy can result in large patient doses if unnecessary grids are not removed (see 'Anti-scatter grids' above) or the radiologist or radiographer does not correctly use or apply their knowledge of the equipment. A simple method of reducing patient dose if imaging a large area containing contrast agent (e.g. barium filled bowel or iodine filled bladder) is to switch off the automatic brightness control to prevent the machine from trying to penetrate the contrast. This simple step can avoid excessive dose to the patient.

## Summary

This chapter aimed to highlight the current radiation protection legislation and suggest practical ways in which radiation protection of children can be improved within the clinical setting. It is not intended to be an exhaustive or prescriptive list of radiation protection measures but a summary of the responsibilities of the radiographer and a revision of easily implemented radiation protection strategies.

# References

1. Graham, D.T. (1996) *Principles of Radiological Physics*, 3rd edn. Churchill Livingstone, London.
2. National Radiation Protection Board (1994) *At A Glance Series – Radiation Protection Standards.* National Radiation Protection Board, Didcot.
3. Statutory Instrument 2000, No. 1059 (2000) The Ionising Radiation (Medical Exposure) Regulations 2000. Stationery Office Limited, London.
4. Statutory Instrument 1999, No. 3232 (1999) The Ionising Radiations Regulations 1999. Stationery Office Limited, London.
5. Kohn, M.M., Moores, B.M, Schibilla, H. *et al.* (eds) (1996) *European Guidelines on Quality Criteria for Diagnostic Radiographic Images in Paediatrics* (EUR 16261 EN). Office for Official Publications of the European Communities, Luxembourg.
6. Grainger, R.G. and Allison, D.J. (1997) *Diagnostic Radiology – A Textbook of Medical Imaging*, 3rd edn. Churchill Livingstone, London.
7. Cook, J.V., Pettet, A., Shah, K. *et al.* (1998) *Guidelines on Best Practice in the X-ray Imaging of Children: A Manual for All X-ray Departments.* Queen Mary's Hospital for Children, The St Helier NHS Trust, Carshalton, Surrey and The Radiological Protection Centre, St George's Healthcare NHS Trust, London.

# Chapter 4
# The chest and upper respiratory tract

Chest radiography is the most frequently performed paediatric plain film examination[1] and may be requested to assist in establishing a preliminary diagnosis, or to monitor the progression of a respiratory condition and assess the effectiveness of any implemented treatment[2]. Despite the relative frequency with which paediatric chest radiography is undertaken, it is still regarded as one of the most clinically challenging examinations to perform adequately and, as a result, many chest radiographs are of reduced image quality, in particular those undertaken on children under 6 years of age[3]. The aim of this chapter is to discuss radiographic technique appropriate to the paediatric chest examination and to consider common technical difficulties that may be encountered in clinical practice. An introduction to paediatric respiratory anatomy and common pathologies has also been included to assist the radiographer in their understanding of paediatric respiratory disease and guide them in their choice of radiographic technique and exposure factors.

## Structural and functional anatomy

### The thorax, lungs and respiratory tract

At birth, the respiratory system is relatively small and under-developed with the normal full-term infant having approximately 25 million alveoli. This number increases to nearly 300 million alveoli by the age of 8 years[4], but after this age the alveoli grow in size rather than number. From this information it can be deduced that a relatively minor respiratory pathology in an 8-year-old child can cause severe respiratory distress in an infant and therefore radiographers should be aware of the varied appearances and clinical presentations of common respiratory disorders.

Growth of the respiratory system is generally faster than growth of the cervical and thoracic spines and therefore anatomical landmarks used to assess an adult chest radiograph are inappropriate for the paediatric patient (e.g. the bifurcation of the trachea, which is seen at the level of the fifth/sixth thoracic vertebra in an adult, lies opposite the third thoracic vertebra in an infant and descends to the level of the fourth thoracic vertebra by approximately 8 years of age). Pelvic growth also affects the size, shape and function of the lungs and thoracic cavity. As the pelvis grows, the abdominal organs descend into the pelvic cavity and reduce the internal pressure the abdomen exerts on the thorax, thereby facilitating flattening of the abdominal walls and lowering of the diaphragm. As a result, the chest shape alters from one that is essentially cylindrical, with the ribs horizontal, to one that is flattened antero-posteriorly with the anterior aspects of the ribs lower than the posterior aspects. This change in chest shape also alters the breathing action of the child from abdominal to diaphragmatic.

### The thymus

The thymus is a lymphoid organ found in the superior aspect of the anterior mediastinum. It is prominent on the chest radiograph of an infant as a result of the thoracic cavity being relatively small; however normal variations in radiographic appearances are common (Figs 4.1a and b). It grows during early childhood to reach a maximum at approximately 15 years of age after which it undergoes regression. It is intensely active during childhood, producing thymus lymphocytes which form part of the human leukocyte antigen mechanism by which the body establishes its system of immunity.

### The heart

The heart is prominent on the chest radiograph of an infant as a result of it lying transversely and occupying approximately 40% of the thoracic cavity. As a consequence, a cardio-thoracic ratio (CTR) of 0.6 is normal for a young child whereas a CTR of 0.5 is considered to be at the upper limit of normal for an adult, assuming a postero-anterior projection of the chest has been undertaken.

## Pathology of the chest and upper respiratory tract

Paediatric respiratory disorders generally result in airway obstruction. Clinical symptoms are dependent upon whether the obstruction is extra-thoracic or intra-thoracic but may include stridor (a harsh sound usually heard on inspiration as a result of a partially obstructed extra-thoracic/upper airway), wheeze (an expiratory noise produced by partial obstruction of the intra-thoracic/lower airway), or crackles/rales (caused by fluid secretions within the alveolar spaces or terminal airways).

### The upper/extra-thoracic airway

#### Adenoidal-tonsillar hypertrophy

The adenoids (nasopharyngeal tonsils) are lymphoid tissue within the nasopharynx concerned with the protection of the upper airway. They are generally small at birth but steadily enlarge until approximately 8 years of age after which they normally regress. Children with hypertrophic (enlarged) adenoids may present clinically with mouth breathing, snoring or possible recurrent otitis

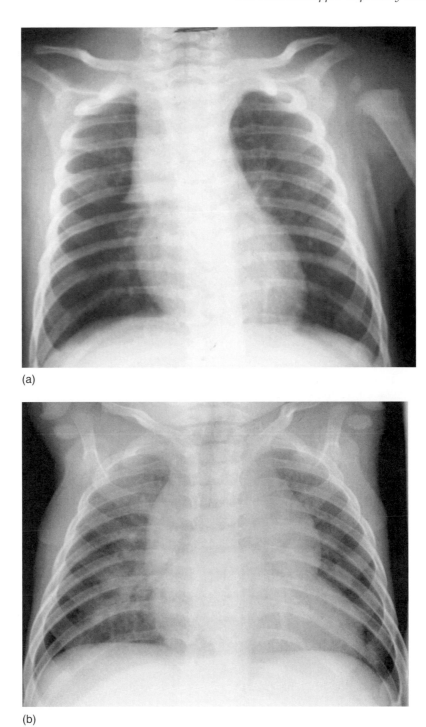

(a)

(b)

**Fig. 4.1** Thymus gland. (a) Normal appearance – sail sign. (b) Normal appearance.

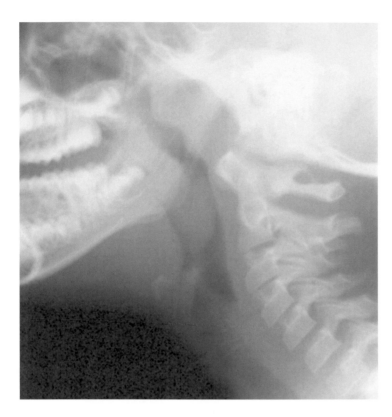

**Fig. 4.2**   Adenoidal-tonsillar hypertrophy. Note the retropharyngeal soft tissue swelling.

media (middle ear infection) as a result of the entrance to the eustachian tube being in close proximity to the nasopharynx. Clinically suspected adenoid hypertrophy can be confirmed on a lateral post-nasal space radiograph[2] (Fig. 4.2).

*Retropharyngeal abscess*

Retropharyngeal abscess is a rare condition presenting in infants (<1 year of age). Clinical symptoms include fever and drooling and, as a result of the swelling within the posterior pharyngeal wall causing upper airway obstruction, the child will typically hold their neck in extension to assist breathing[2]. A lateral soft tissue neck radiograph taken with the neck held in extension is indicated if a retropharyngeal abscess is suspected and if positive this will demonstrate air within the swollen retropharyngeal tissues (Figs 4.3 and 4.4). A contrast enhanced computerised tomography (CT) examination will confirm the diagnosis[5].

*Laryngomalacia*

Laryngomalacia is a relatively common condition that generally presents during the neonatal period as inspiratory stridor. The condition occurs as a result of the epiglottis and arytenoid cartilages collapsing on inspiration and it is usually self-limiting with symptoms disappearing by approximately 2 years of age. The investigative examination of choice is microlaryngobronchoscopy, although

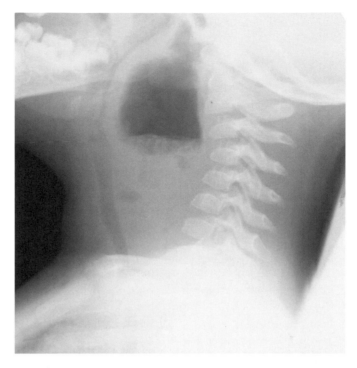

**Fig. 4.3**   Lateral soft tissue neck demonstrating large retropharyngeal abscess.

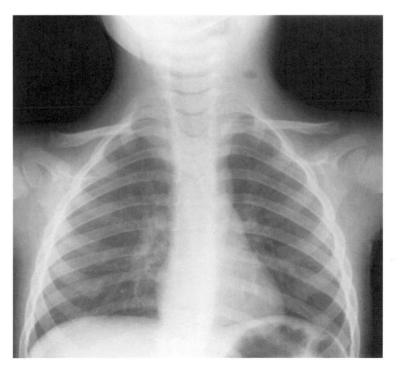

**Fig. 4.4**   Chest radiograph demonstrating gas in a retropharyngeal abscess above the left apex.

ultrasound may also be useful to evaluate pharyngeal anatomy and function. Plain film radiography is NOT indicated.

### Subglottic stenosis

Subglottic stenosis may occur congenitally in infants with Down's syndrome as a result of a narrow larynx. However, it is seen more commonly as a consequence of prolonged endotracheal intubation in premature infants (Figs 4.5 and 4.6). Clinical symptoms include stridor and evidence of respiratory distress. Endoscopic evaluation is the investigation of choice and plain film radiography is NOT indicated.

### Croup (acute infectious laryngotracheobronchitis)

Croup is a combination of stridor, 'barking' cough and respiratory distress as a result of upper airway obstruction, and usually occurs as a consequence of a viral infection in children between the ages of 6 months and 3 years. A definitive diagnosis can normally be made following clinical examination and plain film radiography is NOT indicated.

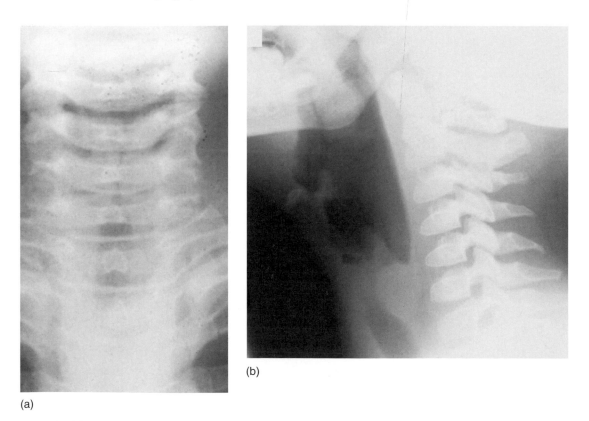

(b)

(a)

**Fig. 4.5**  (a) and (b) Subglottic stenosis. Note the typical 'wine bottle'-shaped airway on antero-posterior (AP) projection.

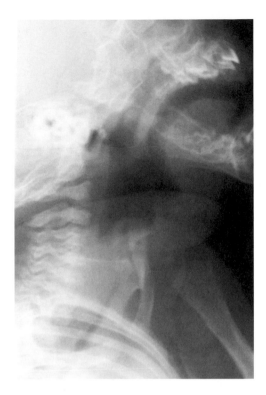

**Fig. 4.6** Sub-glottic stenosis following aggressive intubation.

### Epiglottitis

Epiglottitis is an inflammatory condition of sudden onset and progression that presents in children between the ages of 2 and 7 years. The child will typically sit forward, open mouthed and drooling and, as this condition is a paediatric emergency, should be transferred to a paediatric intensive care unit where investigative laryngoscopy will be undertaken to confirm the clinical diagnosis. Lateral neck radiographs are NOT indicated.

## The lower/intra-thoracic airway

### Asthma

Asthma is an umbrella term for a variety of paediatric chest conditions that result in a persistent or episodic wheeze, possibly associated with a cough. Symptoms typically present in children over the age of 3 years and are more common in the winter months, due to an increase in viruses, and in autumn/spring as a consequence of pollen.

A child known to suffer from asthma does not require radiographic examination with each episode. However, a chest radiograph is indicated if other respiratory conditions are suspected (e.g. pneumothorax, pneumonia or atelectasis). Radiographically, patients with asthma may have a normal chest radiograph therefore supporting the view that asthma is a clinical diagnosis. Alternatively,

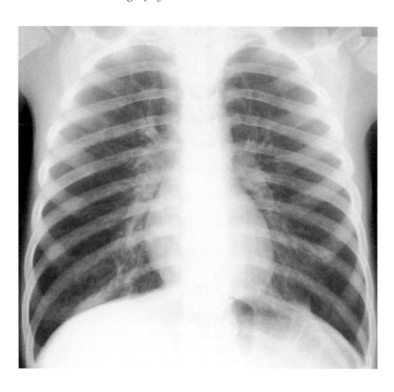

**Fig. 4.7**   Asthma – minimal hyperinflation.

evidence of generalised hyperinflation (flattening of the diaphragm), pneumo-mediastinum and atelectasis may be seen (Fig. 4.7).

*Tracheo-oesophageal fistula*

A tracheo-oesophageal fistula is a variation of oesophageal atresia that presents during the neonatal period (see Chapter 6). Radiographic identification of the site of atresia can be made following the insertion of a radio-opaque feeding tube into the oesophagus. This tube will 'curl' at the site of the atresia and a single antero-posterior projection of the upper abdomen, chest and pharyngeal region should be undertaken. Air identified within the stomach on this projection suggests the presence of a distal fistula. Presentation of oesophageal atresia outside the neonatal period is unusual but may occur with an undiagnosed H-type fistula where the patient presents with repeated chest infections. In these circumstances, a fluoroscopic contrast examination will confirm the diagnosis.

*Bronchiolitis*

Bronchiolitis is the commonest lower respiratory tract infection of infancy with the peak age at presentation being 3 months[2,6]. Clinical symptoms include fever, cough, wheeze and tachypnoea. A plain film radiograph of the chest will display marked hyperinflation of the lungs and possible areas of peribronchial thickening and consolidation.

*Pneumonia*

Pneumonia is the inflammation of the pulmonary tissue[7] and it predominantly presents in children under 5 years of age following a viral infection, although bacterial pneumonia may occur. Clinical symptoms are non-specific but include fever, wheeze and cough. Radiographic appearances are dependent upon the aetiology with viral infections causing air trapping, seen as hyperinflation on the chest radiograph (Fig. 4.8), and bacterial pneumonia displaying radiographic signs of lobar consolidation and pleural effusion (Figs 4.9 and 4.10).

*Bronchiectasis*

Bronchiectasis is defined as the chronic, irreversible dilation and distortion of the bronchi caused by inflammatory destruction of the muscular and elastic components of the bronchial walls[8]. It may be congenital or acquired but usually results from a longstanding localised bronchial infection. Plain film chest radiography is generally insensitive and seldom demonstrates the anatomic distribution of the disease unless the condition is severe when dilated bronchioles will appear as parallel densities (tram lines). Atelectasis may also be seen in severe cases and high-resolution computerised tomography (CT) may be considered to assess the extent and severity of the disease (Fig. 4.11).

*Pulmonary tuberculosis*

Tuberculosis is an infection caused by *Mycobacterium tuberculosis* and, although it is relatively uncommon, incidences of tuberculosis are increasing throughout the world. In the UK, tuberculosis is associated particularly with the immigrant population (especially from Asia, Africa and Latin America), the homeless, the elderly and the immunosuppressed (e.g. people with AIDS). In children, tuberculosis infection is typically due to prolonged and close contact with an individual having active and untreated disease.

The radiographic appearances of pulmonary tuberculosis are varied and dependent upon the age of the child. Progressive pulmonary tuberculosis most commonly occurs during infancy as a result of the primary infection not being contained, and subsequently progresses to bronchopneumonia, lobar pneumonia (usually middle or lower lobe) and cavitation. In contrast, primary pulmonary tuberculosis in older infants and children is usually an asymptomatic illness with minimal abnormalities demonstrated on the chest radiograph, while adolescent infection will follow more closely the typical adult appearances with upper lobe opacification and possible cavitation. Widespread haematogenous dissemination of tuberculosis following primary infection is uncommon and is normally restricted to children under 2 years of age[9] (Fig. 4.12).

*AIDS (acquired immunodeficiency syndrome)*

The lungs are a common site of infection in the immunocompromised child and consequently over 50% of AIDS-related paediatric mortalities have pulmonary disease[5] (Fig. 4.13). The radiographic appearances of AIDS-related paediatric

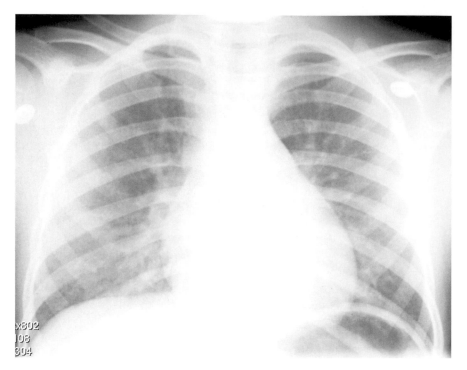

**Fig. 4.8** Viral pneumonia.

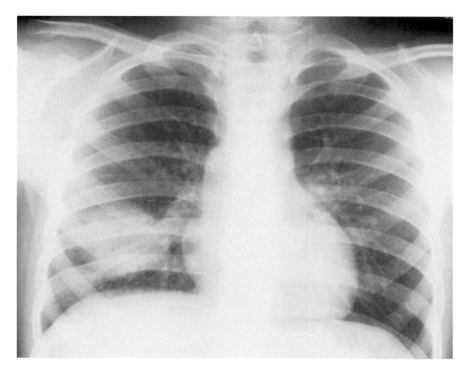

**Fig. 4.9** Bacterial pneumonia giving rise to the appearance of consolidation in the right lung.

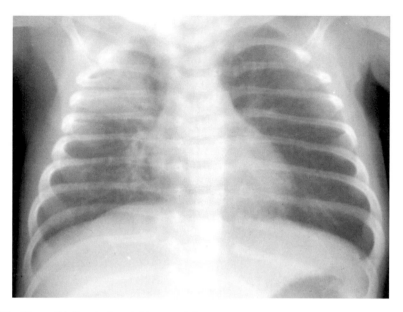

**Fig. 4.10** Consolidation in the right upper lobe.

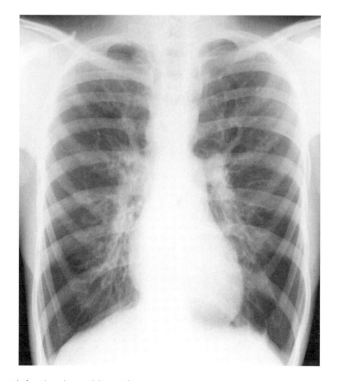

**Fig. 4.11** Post-infection bronchiectasis.

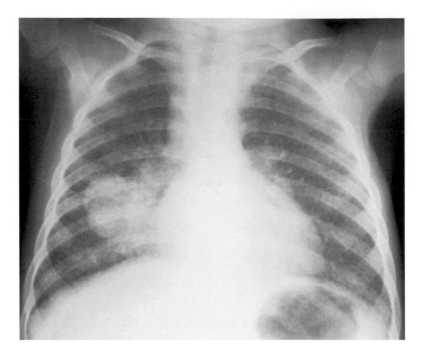

**Fig. 4.12**  Primary tuberculosis.

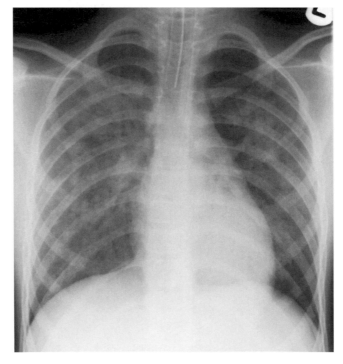

**Fig. 4.13**  Pneumocystis pneumonia associated with immunosuppressed patients.

pneumonia are variable and non-specific, and therefore the accurate diagnosis of the underlying cause of pneumonia requires further invasive investigation (e.g. lung biospy).

## The chest wall and pleura

### Scoliosis

When severe, scoliosis may result in respiratory dysfunction as a consequence of a marked curvature of the thoracic spine and associated chest wall deformity restricting normal thoracic inspiratory and expiratory movement. Significant loss of inspiratory capacity may lead to pulmonary hypertension, recurrent infection, atelectasis and respiratory insufficiency.

### Pectus excavatum

Pectus excavatum (funnel chest) is depression of the sternum and results in a reduction in the antero-posterior diameter of the thoracic cavity (Fig. 4.14). As a consequence, there is insufficient room for the heart to lie in its normal position

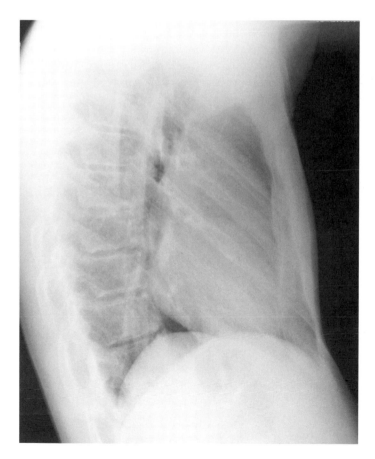

**Fig. 4.14** Pectus excavatum resulting in compression of the antero-posterior (AP) diameter of the chest.

behind the sternum and it is commonly displaced towards the left, giving the impression of cardiac enlargement with possible associated right middle lobe pathology if the right heart border is unclear[10]. If not identified clinically at the time of examination, pectus excavatum can be suspected radiographically if the anterior ribs are seen sloping steeply on the postero-anterior projection of the chest.

*Pneumothorax*

Pneumothorax is defined as air within the pleural space[7] that results in total or partial collapse of the lung. It may occur spontaneously, particularly in tall, thin, male adolescents, or as a result of trauma, medical intervention or as a consequence of another respiratory condition (e.g. asthma, cystic fibrosis) (Fig. 4.15). Patients with a pneumothorax will present clinically with chest pain, dyspnoea and cyanosis. Plain film radiography of the chest will display increased radio-opacification of the deflated lung, evidence of the lung edge medial to the wall of the thorax and increased radiolucency lateral to the lung. Treatment is typically by insertion of a chest drain to remove the air from the pleural space and allow the lung to re-inflate. A small pneumothorax will generally resolve without medical intervention.

A tension pneumothorax (Fig. 4.16) is an acute surgical emergency and usually occurs as a result of traumatic injury to the chest wall. The puncture wound acts like a valve allowing air into the pleural cavity on inspiration but closing to prevent air escaping on expiration thereby resulting in increasing pressure within the pleural cavity and compression of the lung and mediastinum. This condition requires immediate surgical intervention and diagnosis is based upon clinical examination. Post-interventional plain film radiography of the chest may be required to assess lung re-expansion.

*Pneumomediastinum*

Pneumomediastinum is the presence of air within the mediastinum (Fig. 4.17). The most common cause of pneumomediastinum in children is asthma and results from alveolar rupture (see Chapter 6).

*Pleural effusion*

Pleural effusion is defined as fluid within the pleural cavity and generally occurs as a reaction to another pathological condition (e.g. congestive heart failure, malignancy, collagen-vascular disease, inflammation or infection of the pleura, and obstruction of lymphatic drainage). It may be identified on an erect chest radiograph (postero-anterior or lateral) as blunting of the costophrenic angles (Fig. 4.18) or, if chest radiography has been performed with the patient supine, as fluid surrounding the lung resulting in increased radiographic opacification. The altered translucency of the lung, which occurs as a result of imaging a pleural effusion in the supine position, may be subtle and therefore, if a pleural effusion

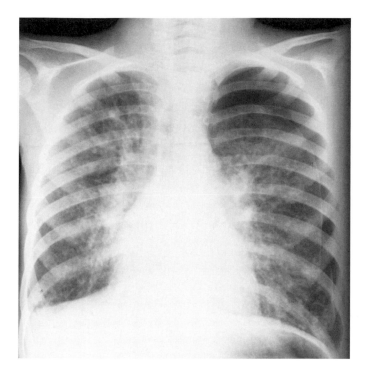

**Fig. 4.15**   Left-sided pneumothorax in a patient with cystic fibrosis.

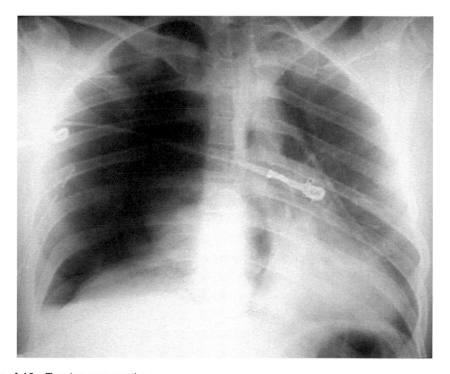

**Fig. 4.16**   Tension pneumothorax.

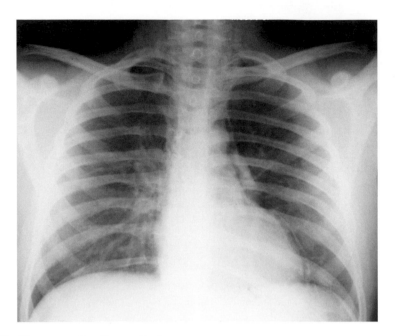

**Fig. 4.17**    Air surrounding the mediastinum.

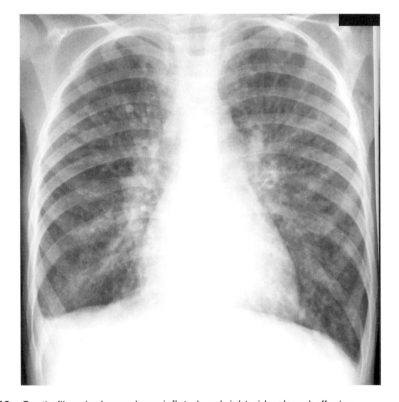

**Fig. 4.18**    Cystic fibrosis. Lungs hyperinflated and right-side pleural effusion.

is suspected, an antero-posterior or postero-anterior projection of the chest with the patient in the decubitus position (affected side down) may be necessary to confirm the diagnosis.

## Cystic fibrosis

Cystic fibrosis is the most common, lethal, genetic disease affecting Caucasians and is reported to be present in 1:2500 live births in the UK[2]. It is a multi-system disease that affects the epithelial cells of all major organs, resulting in changes to their absorptive and secretory characteristics. Cystic fibrosis of the respiratory epithelium leads to dehydration of the airway secretions and results in airway obstruction and chronic bronchial infection (cough, sputum production, hyper-inflation and bronchiectasis). The chest radiograph is the primary method of radiological evaluation[5] and, in the early stages of the disease, will display signs of airway thickening and hyperinflation (Fig. 4.18). Cystic fibrosis results in premature mortality, the median survival age being 27 years, and the severity of the pulmonary disease is often an influential factor.

## Pulmonary neoplasm

Primary tumours of the respiratory tract are rare in children. However, metastatic spread from osseous or abdominal malignancies (Wilms' tumour, neuroblastoma, osteosarcoma) is relatively common and spiral CT is the imaging modality of choice to assess the extent of pulmonary metastatic disease.

## Atelectasis

The term atelectasis is defined as 'airless lung' and is synonymous with the collapse of a lobe or lung. Atelectasis occurs as a consequence of respiratory obstruction and should be suspected if, on the postero-anterior radiograph, there is an area of increased opacification associated with loss of clarity of the mediastinal, cardiac or diaphragmatic outlines and, on the right, movement of the horizontal fissure (Figs 4.19–4.22). Right upper lobe collapse is seen predominantly in children.

## Foreign body aspiration

Foreign body aspiration is a relatively common paediatric event that typically presents between the ages of 9 months and 3 years. A foreign body lodged within a main bronchus results in persistent hyperinflation of the affected lung or lobe as a result of the 'ball valve effect' where air is allowed to enter the lung on inspiration but is obstructed and unable to leave the lung on expiration. As in adults, inspired foreign bodies are usually identified in the right main bronchus as a result of it being wider and more vertical. However, in infants, the tracheal bifurcation is more central and foreign bodies may be seen equally in the left and right main bronchi (Fig. 4.23). Unless the foreign body is radio-opaque, plain film

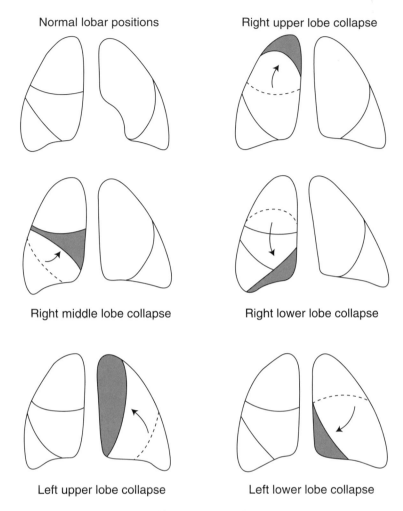

**Fig. 4.19**   Diagrammatic illustration of lobar atelectasis.

radiographic evidence is initially limited to recognising subtle changes in the radioluceny of the hyperinflated lung when compared with the opposite lung (Fig. 4.24). Patients with an unidentified foreign body will present several days later with a persistent cough and signs of systemic illness as a result of a pulmonary infection at the sight of the foreign body obstruction. This infection will not resolve unless the foreign body is removed and therefore a persistent, unresolving pneumonia in a young child should raise clinical suspicion of foreign body aspiration.

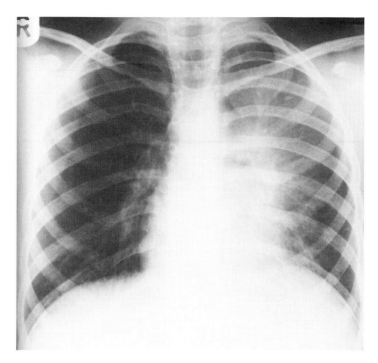

**Fig. 4.20** Left upper lobe collapse. Note loss of the left heart border.

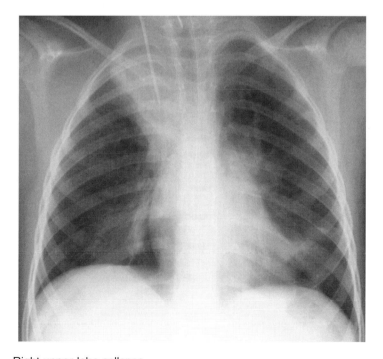

**Fig. 4.21** Right upper lobe collapse.

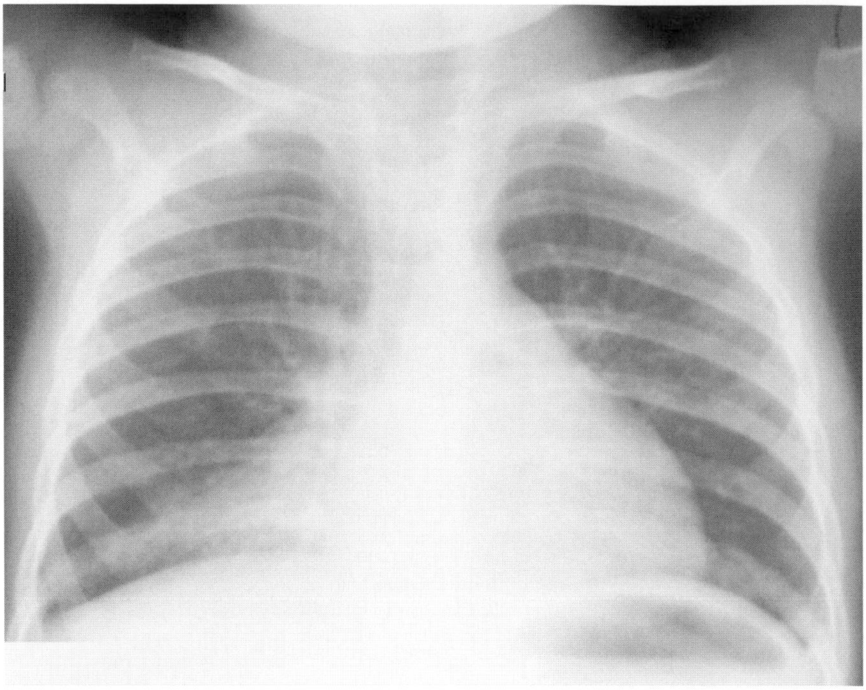

(a)

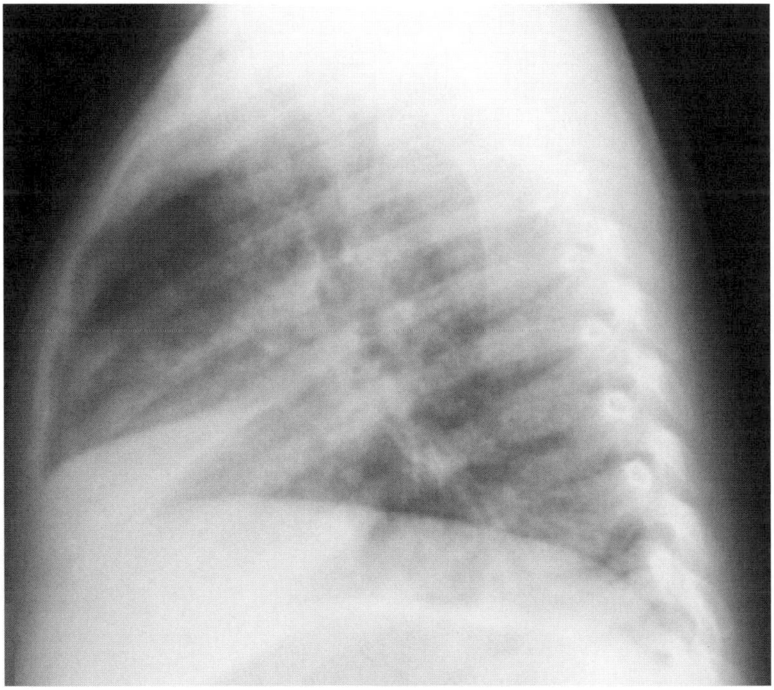

(b)

**Fig. 4.22**   (a) and (b) Right middle lobe collapse confirmed on lateral. Note loss of right heart border on antero-posterior projection.

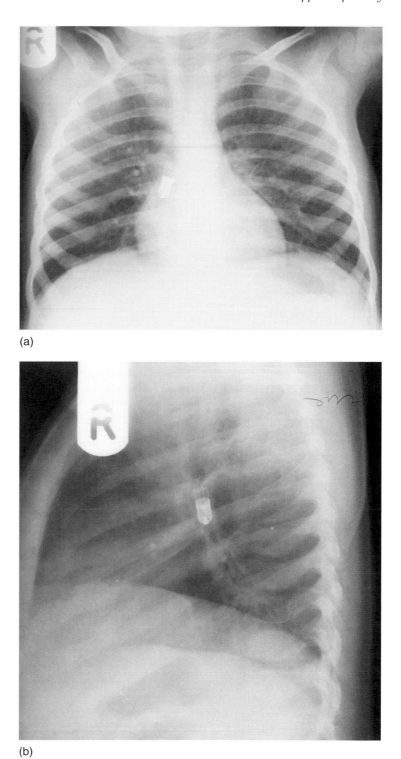

(a)

(b)

**Fig. 4.23** (a) and (b) Inhaled foreign body. Note the torch bulb in the right main bronchus.

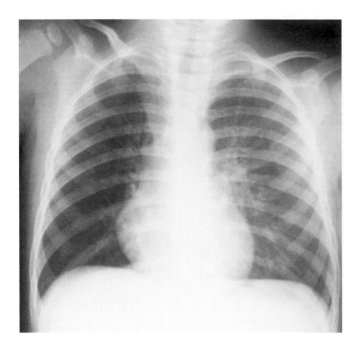

**Fig. 4.24**  Radiolucent foreign body in right main bronchus. Note the increased radiolucency of the right lung as a result of air trapping.

# Radiographic technique for the chest and upper respiratory tract

Plain film radiography remains the first-line examination for the majority of respiratory conditions. However, alternative imaging modalities may be used to assess the extent of a disease or confirm a diagnosis (Box 4.1 and Fig. 4.25).

**Box 4.1**  The role of imaging in the determination of chest disease

*Fluoroscopy*:  Provides dynamic images which may be useful to clarify the presence of a suspected pathology visualised on plain films (e.g. obstructive emphysema). Its use is decreasing due to the recognition of high patient doses and the development of other imaging modalities.

*Ultrasound*:  Of little value for the respiratory system but extremely useful in the investigation of cardiac and mediastinal pathology. It can be used for guided needle aspiration of pleural effusions.

*Computed tomography (CT)*:  Second-line imaging modality after plain films. It provides good contrast and spatial resolution of lung parenchyma, mediastinum and bony structures but has the disadvantage that sedation is often required due to the length of examination.

*Magnetic resonance imaging (MRI)*:  Useful for examining the mediastinum and the chest wall but has the disadvantage that young children will require sedation and frequently general anaesthetic due to the relatively long imaging times.

*Scintigraphy*:  Of value in the investigation of pulmonary embolisms and bony pathology (e.g. occult rib fractures or metastatic deposits).

*Angiography*:  Used for cardio-vascular studies. Its use is on the decline as a result of improvements in ultrasound and MRI but it has the advantage of facilitating interventional procedures.

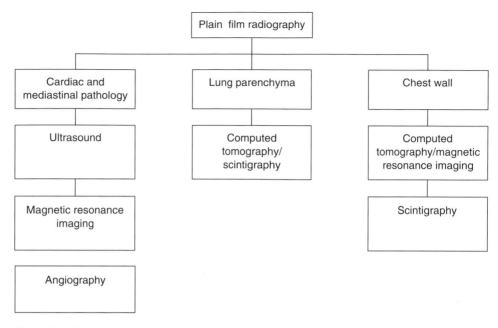

**Fig. 4.25** Chest imaging decision tree.

**Table 4.1** Guide to common practice for paediatric chest radiography.

| Age (approximately) | Projection | Patient position |
|---|---|---|
| Under 3 months | Antero-posterior | Supine |
| 3 months to 4 years | Antero-posterior | Erect |
| 4 years and older | Postero-anterior | Erect |

## Choice of projection

There is no difference in the diagnostic value of an antero-posterior (AP) projection compared to the postero-anterior (PA) projection of the chest in a child less than 4 years of age as the thoracic cage is essentially cylindrical in young children and magnification of mediastinal organs is insignificant[11]. However, the AP projection is associated with a higher radiation dose to the developing breast, sternum and thyroid, and radiographers should take this into consideration when choosing the radiographic projection.

In children under 4 years of age, the AP projection is often preferred due to ease of positioning, immobilisation and maintenance of patient communication. Young children like to see what is going on around them and positioning for an AP projection allows the child to watch the radiographer. A disadvantage of the AP projection is the likelihood of lordosis but this can be prevented by careful technique. Table 4.1 provides a guide to common practice in paediatric chest radiography.

It is important to ensure that whatever protocol is adopted, it is consistently applied within the imaging department to ensure consistent radiographic results are achieved. This is particularly important if the child's condition is being monitored radiographically as subtle radiographic changes in their condition may be difficult to interpret if the technical (positioning) factors are inconsistent. The following descriptions of radiographic positioning are provided as a guide and may be modified depending upon equipment and accessories available.

### Antero-posterior (supine)

The patient is positioned supine with the median sagittal plane at 90° to the image receptor. A 15° foam pad is placed under the upper chest and shoulders to prevent lordosis (Fig. 4.26). The chin is raised and the arms are flexed and held on either side of the head to prevent rotation (Figs 4.27 and 4.28). Sandbags and lead rubber are placed over the hips and legs to provide immobilisation of the

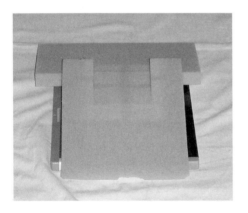

**Fig. 4.26** A 15° foam pad for use in chest radiography. The cut out area helps to prevent the chin obscuring the upper chest.

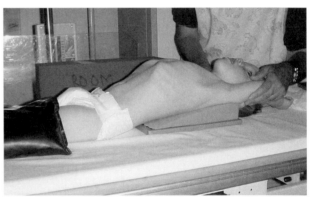

**Fig. 4.27** Poor supine chest technique. Note that although a 15° pad has been used, the extension of the patient's arms will still result in a lordotic radiograph.

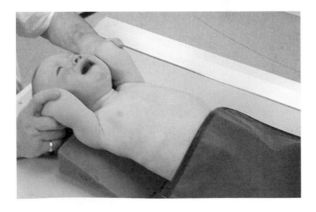

**Fig. 4.28** Correct supine chest technique. Note the use of a 15° foam pad and arms positioned with elbows flexed to prevent hyperextension of the spine and lordosis.

legs or alternatively, the legs may be held at the knees by the accompanying guardian.

The primary beam should be centred to the area of interest thereby ensuring that effective collimation can be applied and dose reduction optimised.

### Antero-posterior (erect)

This projection can be performed with the patient standing or seated erect. For younger children, correct positioning and immobilisation are easier to maintain with the child seated. It is important when seating a child to ensure that the legs are not extended level with the buttocks, as this will accentuate lordosis[12] (Fig. 4.29). Instead, a young child should be seated on a sponge/box thereby lowering the level of the legs and reducing lordosis (Fig. 4.30).

The patient is positioned initially with the posterior aspect of the chest in contact with a cassette. A 15° foam pad is then placed behind the upper chest and shoulders to prevent lordosis. The chin is raised and the arms are flexed and held on either side of the head by a suitably protected guardian to prevent rotation (Fig. 4.31).

The primary beam is centred to the middle of the area of interest and collimated to within the area of the cassette.

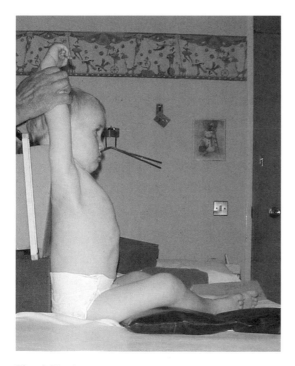

**Fig. 4.29** Incorrect technique. Arms extended and legs at the same level as the hips. Note the child appears lordotic.

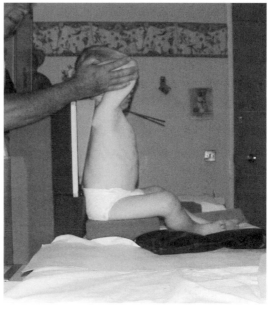

**Fig. 4.30** Correct technique. Note the child is seated on a foam sponge and a 15° pad is placed behind the chest to reduce lordosis. The arms are held flexed at the side of the head by a suitably protected guardian.

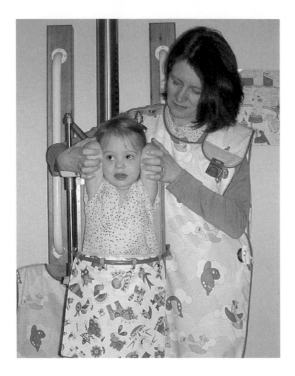

**Fig. 4.31**   Antero-posterior (AP) chest technique on a young ambulant child. Note the guardian holds the child's flexed elbows at the side of the head to ensure there is no rotation. The AP projection allows the child to watch what is happening around them and reduces apprehension.

### Postero-anterior (erect)

This projection can be performed with the patient standing or seated. The patient is positioned with the anterior aspect of the chest in contact with a cassette and their arms encircling it (Fig. 4.32a). Both shoulders should touch the cassette to ensure that there is no rotation. The cassette is positioned to include both apices and the patient's chin is rested on the cassette top. It is often easier for a young child to maintain this position rather than the more traditional position of the hands being placed on the back of the hips. However, if you are reasonably satisfied that the child will maintain the adult position then this should be adopted as it is more likely to provide clearance of the scapulae from the chest (Fig. 4.32b).

The primary beam is centred to the middle of the area of interest and collimated to within the area of the cassette.

## Radiographic assessment criteria for antero-posterior/ postero-anterior projections of the chest

### Area of interest to be included on the radiograph

The radiograph should include the whole of the chest from, and including, the first rib to the costophrenic angles inferiorly and the outer margins of the ribs laterally.

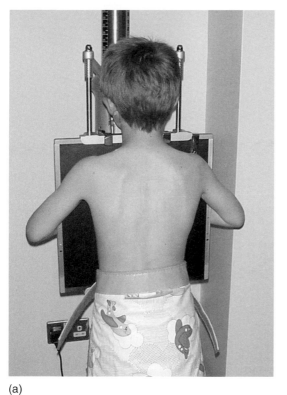

(a)

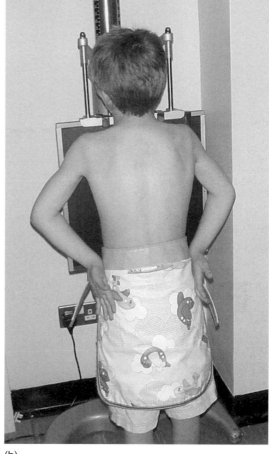

(b)

**Fig. 4.32**   (a) and (b) Postero-anterior projections of the chest.

### Rotation

The chest of a young child is more cylindrical than that of an adult and therefore a small amount of rotation will lead to the appearance of significant asymmetry. Due to difficulties visualising the medial ends of the clavicles in young children, rotation is better judged using the anterior ribs, which should be of equal length and symmetrically positioned with respect to the vertebral column. Minimising patient rotation is essential as many pathological conditions may be simulated as a result of rotation (e.g. hyperlucent lung, enlarged cardiac outline) (Fig. 4.33).

### Lordosis

Lordosis is a common technical fault when performing antero-posterior chest radiography and may be resolved by placing a 15° pad behind the patient's

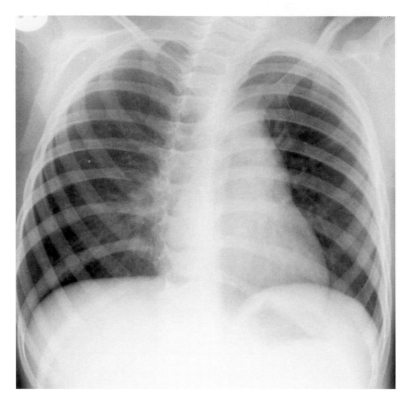

**Fig. 4.33**  Rotated postero-anterior projection. Note the unusual cardiac outline and the asymmetric appearance of the anterior ribs.

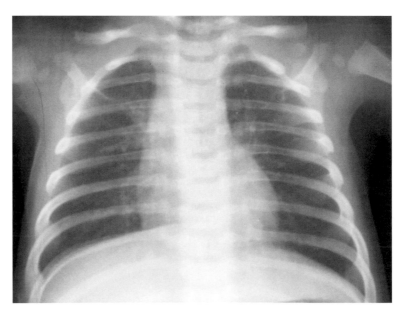

**Fig. 4.34**  A lordotic antero-posterior projection. Note that the anterior ribs are horizontal.

shoulders and by ensuring that the arms are not hyperextended. Radiographically, lordosis can be identified when the anterior ribs appear horizontal or are angled cranially to lie above the posterior ribs. The altered position of the clavicles is not an accurate indication of lordosis in children as clavicular position changes with shoulder movement (Fig. 4.34).

## Respiration

Failure to achieve satisfactory inspiration is a common problem when radiographing children. In young children, the phase of respiration can be assessed by observing the rise and fall of the abdomen. It must be remembered that the shape of the paediatric chest alters with growth and therefore the assessment of adequate inspiration by rib counting also changes (Table 4.2). Adequate inspiration is important in order to visualise the lung fields clearly and to avoid the impression of cardiomegaly and prominent pulmonary vasculature[13].

**Table 4.2**   A guide to the assessment of inspiration on a chest radiograph.

| Age of child | Optimum inspiration |
| --- | --- |
| 0–3 years | 6 anterior ribs, 8 posterior ribs |
| 3–7 years | 6 anterior ribs, 9 posterior ribs |
| 8 years + | 6 anterior ribs, 10 posterior ribs |

## Exposure

A correctly exposed radiograph should demonstrate pulmonary vessels in the central two-thirds of the lung fields without evidence of blurring. The trachea and major bronchi should also be visible as should the intervertebral disc spaces of the lower thoracic spine through the heart.

## Artefacts

Care should be taken to avoid artefacts on children's clothing (e.g. transfers on vests and T-shirts) and hair should be moved away from the area of interest (Fig. 4.35).

# Supplementary radiographic projections of the chest and upper respiratory tract

## Lateral chest

The lateral chest should not be undertaken routinely and should only be performed if referral criteria satisfy departmental protocols for a lateral projection or following discussion with a radiologist.

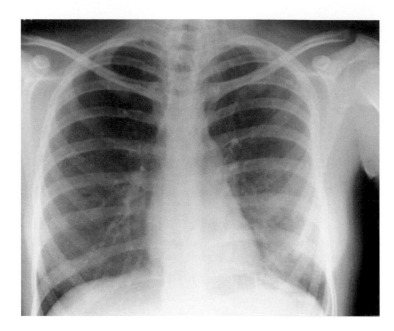

**Fig. 4.35** Hair artefact visible as 'streaking' lateral to the mediastinal contour.

Lateral chest radiography is often easier to perform on young children if they are seated. The child sits or stands with the side under investigation closest to an appropriately sized cassette. The cassette is positioned to include the whole of the chest. The patient's chin is raised and the arms are flexed at the elbow and held on either side of the head by a suitably protected guardian to prevent rotation. An older child may prefer to maintain this position unaided (Fig. 4.36).

The primary beam is centred to the middle of the area of interest and collimated to within the area of the cassette.

*Radiographic assessment criteria of lateral chest*

The posterior aspects of the ribs should be superimposed and the vertebrae should be seen without rotation. The radiograph should include the whole of the chest from the apices to the diaphragm.

## Lateral decubitus (antero-posterior)

The lateral decubitus projection is useful when a horizontal beam projection is required and the patient cannot be positioned erect. If a pneumothorax is suspected, the projection should be undertaken with the affected side uppermost while if a pleural effusion is suspected, the affected side should be lowermost.

The child lies on their side on top of rectangular foam pads of suitable length to allow the whole of the chest to be visualised on the resultant radiograph. The cassette is placed behind the child and the child is positioned such that the median sagittal plane is 90° to the cassette. The child's knees are flexed to provide stability and the arms are flexed and placed in front of their head. An appropriately protected adult may hold the cassette and the patient's hands if required.

*Radiographic assessment criteria of lateral decubitus*

The appropriate area of interest to be included is from the apices, including all of the first rib, to the costophrenic angles and the outer margins of the ribs laterally.

## Lateral soft tissue neck

This projection may be required to investigate a suspected foreign body or soft tissue swelling. The patient is seated so that the median sagittal plane is parallel to the cassette. The chin is raised and the head and neck are carefully positioned to reduce lateral rotation. A rectangular sponge placed between the cassette and the child's head may assist in maintaining the position and with immobilisation. The arms are relaxed at the side of the patient and, in young children, it may be advantageous for the guardian to be seated in front of the child, holding the arms and encouraging them to maintain the position. For imaging young children exposure should be made during inspiration. However,

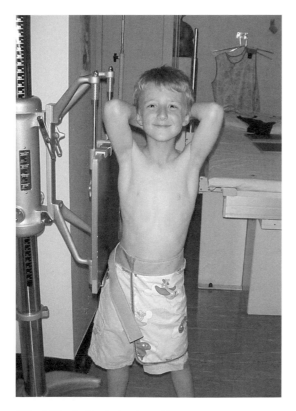

**Fig. 4.36**  Lateral chest position.

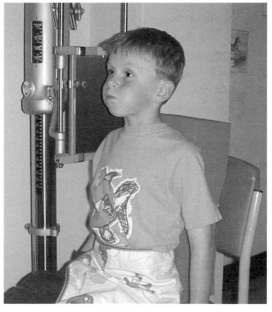

**Fig. 4.37**  Lateral soft tissue neck. The child is seated with their hands placed by their sides. A long rectangular sponge is placed behind the patient's back to assist in immobilisation. This patient is performing the Val salva manoeuvre.

older children may be able to successfully perform the Val salva manoeuvre (forced expiration against a closed glottis) (Fig. 4.37). The horizontal beam is centred midway between the sternal notch and the mastoid process.

*Radiographic assessment criteria of lateral soft tissue neck*

The mandibular rami should be superimposed and the pharynx and trachea down to the level of the thoracic inlet should be included and outlined with air.

## Post-nasal space

A well-collimated lateral projection of the post-nasal space will demonstrate soft tissue encroachment onto the air-filled pharynx (e.g. enlarged adenoids).

The patient sits facing an 18 × 24 cm cassette. The head is then rotated so that the median sagittal plane is parallel to the cassette. The chin is raised and the neck should be straight. Immobilisation is achieved by ensuring that both hands hold the erect cassette holder (Fig. 4.38). For examination of a young child, a suitably protected guardian may need to hold the head still. Exposure should be made with the patient's mouth closed on gentle inspiration. The primary beam should be centred over the middle of the mandibular ramus and to the centre of the film.

**Note**:  Careful collimation should be undertaken to avoid irradiation of the thyroid gland and the lens of the eyes.

*Radiographic assessment criteria of post-nasal space*

The mandibular rami should be superimposed and the nasopharynx clearly outlined with air.

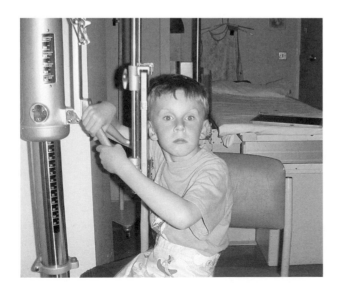

**Fig. 4.38**  Lateral post-nasal space projection. Note the child's arms are positioned around the erect cassette holder to assist in immobilisation.

**Table 4.3** Exposure factors: guidelines for the antero-posterior and postero-anterior chest projection[14].

| Age (years) | Focal spot | Kilovoltage (kV) | mAs | FFD[a] (cm) | Relative screen/ film speed | Grid | AEC[b] |
|---|---|---|---|---|---|---|---|
| <1 | Fine | 60 | 2 | 150 | 400–800 | No | No |
| 1–4 | Broad | 75 | 2 | 150 | 400–800 | No | No |
| 4–10 | Broad | 75 | 4 | 150 | 400–800 | Yes | No |
| 10+ | Broad | 80–120 (dependent on size) | AEC | 150–180 | 400–800 | Yes/No (dependent on size) | Yes |

[a] Focus-to-film distance.
[b] Automatic exposure control.

## Exposure factors and radiation protection

The European Guidelines[14] recommend a fast film screen combination, 400–800 speed class, for use in paediatric chest radiography combined with an exposure time of less than 10 ms to reduce the risk of recorded movement unsharpness.

The use of automatic exposure control (AEC) is not recommended for infants and small children due to the relatively large size of the chamber compared to the area of interest and the difficulty of positioning the chamber to an appropriate anatomical area.

The kilovoltage (kV) selected is influenced by the size of the child. A relatively high kV should be used to reduce the radiation dose (Table 4.3). If difficulties in using high kV are encountered as a result of being unable to set sufficiently low mAs values then increasing the filtration within the tube is advocated. This will reduce tube output per mAs thereby allowing tube potential to be increased for infant examinations[15]. Additional filtration will also reduce the amount of low energy photons within the radiation beam and therefore assist in the reduction of patient dose. Additional filtration of up to 1 mm aluminium plus 0.1 or 0.2 mm copper or equivalent is recommended[14].

The use of an anti-scatter grid or Bucky is not appropriate for chest radiography on small children. However, it may be used when imaging large adolescents.

Table 4.3 outlines the typical exposure factor combinations for an antero-posterior or postero-anterior chest projection across a range of paediatric ages. These examples assume that additional filtration has been added to the x-ray tube as recommended by the European Guidelines[14].

## Summary

Although frequently undertaken, many radiographers are still uncomfortable performing paediatric chest examinations and it is hoped that, by providing a description of suitable techniques, including associated radiographic assessment criteria and common chest pathologies, the radiographer will be able to improve not only their technical ability, but also their understanding of paediatric pulmonary diseases.

# References

1. Haller, J.O. and Slovis, T.L. (1995) *Pediatric Radiology*, 2nd edn. Springer, London.
2. Campbell, A.G.M. and McIntosh, N. (1998) *Forfar and Arneil's Textbook of Pediatrics*, 5th edn. Churchill Livingstone, Edinburgh.
3. Engelmann, D., Dutting, T., Wunsch, R. and Troger, J. (2001) Quality of ambulatory thoracic radiography in the child – a pilot study. *Radiologe* **41** (5), 442–6.
4. Sinclair, D. and Dangerfield, P. (1998) *Human Growth After Birth*, 6th edn. Oxford University Press, Oxford.
5. Grainger, R.G., Allison, D.J., Adam, A. and Dixon, A.K. (2001) *Grainger and Allison's Diagnostic Radiology – A Textbook of Medical Imaging*, 4th edn. Churchill Livingstone, London.
6. Behrman, R.E. and Kliegman, R.M. (eds) (1994) *Essentials of Pediatrics*, 2nd edn. WB Saunders Company, London.
7. Armstrong, P., Wilson, A.G., Dee, P. and Hansell, D.M. (2000) *Imaging of Diseases of the Chest*, 3rd edn. Mosby, London.
8. George, R.B., Light, R.W., Matthay, M.A. and Matthay, R.A. (2000) *Chest Medicine, Essentials of Pulmonary and Critical Care Medicine*, 4th edn. Lippincott Williams & Wilkins, Philadelphia.
9. Juhl, J.H., Crummy, A.B. and Kuhlman, J.E. (1998) *Essentials of Radiologic Imaging*, 7th edn. Lippincott-Raven, New York.
10. Schlesinger, A.E. (1998) Pitfalls in the interpretation of pediatric chest and airway radiographs. *Current Problems in Diagnostic Radiology* **27** (3), 73–101.
11. Blickman, J.G. (1994) *Pediatric Radiology: The Requisites*. Mosby, London.
12. Gyll, C. and Blake, N. (1986) *Paediatric Diagnostic Imaging*. William Heinemann Medical Books, London.
13. Carty, H., Shaw, D., Brunelle, F. and Kendall, B. (eds) (1994) *Imaging Children*. Churchill Livingstone, London.
14. Kohn, M.M., Moores, B.M., Schibilla, H. *et al.* (eds) (1996) *European Guidelines on Quality Criteria for Diagnostic Radiographic Images in Paediatrics* (EUR 16261 EN). Office for Official Publications of the European Communities, Luxembourg.
15. Mooney, R. and Thomas, P.S. (1998) Dose reduction in paediatric X-ray departments following optimisation of radiographic technique. *British Journal of Radiology* **71**, 852–60.

# Chapter 5
# The abdomen

Radiography has a significant role to play in the investigation of the paediatric abdomen, particularly in the identification of gastrointestinal and genitourinary pathology. However, the use of ionising radiation for imaging the paediatric abdomen is increasingly being questioned and radiographers must ensure that plain film radiography is justified as there are an increasing number of clinical presentations for which plain film radiography is no longer appropriate as the first-line imaging investigation.

## Structural and functional anatomy

The abdomen is defined by the diaphragm superiorly and the pelvic inlet inferiorly. Most abdominal radiography, however, relates to the gastrointestinal and genitourinary tracts and these anatomical systems extend beyond these boundaries.

### Gastrointestinal system

The gastrointestinal system extends from the mouth superiorly to the anal opening and includes the buccal cavity, the pharynx, the oesophagus, the stomach, and the small and large bowel.

At birth, the tongue lies wholly within the mouth and during the first 4 or 5 years of life, the posterior part descends with the larynx to form part of the anterior wall of the pharynx. Before the tongue and larynx descend, their high position allows the child to breathe freely while fluid passes down on either side of the epiglottis and uvula into the oesphagus[1]. The stomach lies horizontally across the upper abdomen at birth and increases its capacity from approximately 30 ml to 500 ml during the first year of life. The remainder of the gastrointestinal tract grows at a slower pace, the small bowel doubling its length between birth and puberty. The small and large bowel are both thin walled at birth due to the underdevelopment of musculature and therefore radiological differentiation in the young infant can be difficult as the characteristic colonic haustrations and small bowel valvulae conniventes may not be apparent. In addition, little of the small bowel lies within the pelvis until after 2 years of age due to the small size of the infant pelvis.

### Genitourinary system

The urinary system lies in the retroperitoneal space and normally comprises bilateral kidneys postero-laterally in the right and left upper abdominal quadrants. Extending from the kidneys bilaterally are the ureters, which open inferiorly into the posterior aspect of the base of the urinary bladder. The urethra extends from the neck of the bladder to the exterior and is longer in the male than in the female.

The kidneys are not fully functional at birth and glomerular filtration within the first year of life is relatively poor[1]. Growth of the kidneys is dependent upon the amount of work they do and evidence for this is the excessive or compensatory growth of one kidney if the contra-lateral kidney fails to function correctly or is removed.

The urinary bladder lies predominantly within the abdomen at birth with relative movement inferiorly as the pelvic cavity enlarges.

The gonads and external genitalia have a slow rate of development during childhood but this increases in adolescence under the influence of gonadotrophic hormones.

The only major organs in the male pelvis at birth are the rectum and the prostate gland. The female pelvis is more crowded containing the rectum, vagina and uterus with the ovaries and bladder lying within the abdominal cavity at the level of the pelvic brim[2,3]. Full descent of the ovaries and bladder into the female pelvis may not occur until as late as the sixth year of life[1] and this warrants consideration when positioning radiation protection devices on a female child.

# Gastrointestinal pathology

Many referrals relating to the paediatric gastrointestinal tract are associated with congenital anomalies and present within the first month of life if not prenatally. Conditions such as bowel atresia, congenital megacolon and malrotation are discussed within Chapter 6 (neonatal radiography). However, some of these abnormalities will present as a functional disturbance after the neonatal period along with other developmental and acquired conditions (e.g. pyloric stenosis). This chapter will cover pathology not specifically associated with the neonatal period.

### Congenital pyloric stenosis

Pyloric stenosis most commonly occurs due to hypertrophy of the pyloric muscle and causes obstruction of the gastric outlet[4]. It is more common in males than females with the classic presentation being non-bilious projectile vomiting and weight loss noted at the routine 6-week postnatal check-up[5]. A clinical diagnosis is possible by palpating an olive-shaped mass to the right of the umbilicus and confirmation can be achieved with sonographic demonstration of a thick hypoechoic ring representing the hypertrophied muscle layer[6]. Reliable diagno-

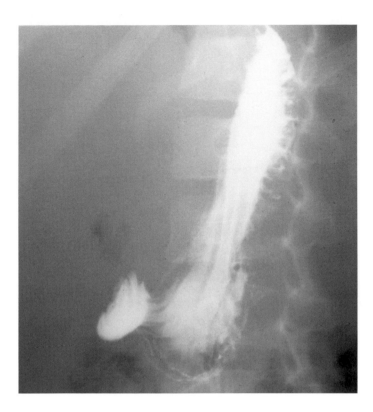

**Fig. 5.1** Pyloric stenosis. The pylorus is enlarged and the duodenal bulb is indented, consistent with hypertrophy.

sis can be achieved with ultrasound even in the absence of a palpable mass and plain film radiography and gastrointestinal contrast studies are NOT routinely indicated (Fig. 5.1).

## *Intussusception*

Although relatively uncommon, intussusception is the most frequent cause of intestinal obstruction in children under 2 years of age[7]. It most commonly presents between 6 and 18 months of age[6].

Although the exact cause is unknown, intussusception occurs when peristalsis becomes irregular and one segment of bowel prolapses into another (Figs. 5.2 and 5.3). The most common site for intussusception is the ileocaecal region where the terminal ileum may 'telescope' into the caecum. The severity of the condition is exacerbated if the blood supply to the prolapsed segment is compromised by associated mesenteric invagination causing blood vessel compression[8].

Ultrasound is the imaging modality of choice to confirm a clinical diagnosis and to guide treatment. However, plain film radiography of the abdomen may also be undertaken depending upon local circumstances and paediatric expertise[5,9,10]. Non-surgical reduction of intussusception can be achieved using an 'air-enema' technique. This is usually performed under fluoroscopic control and may be successful in up to 85% of cases[11]. This procedure is contraindicated in the presence of pneumoperitoneum or when clinical evidence suggests peritonitis[8]

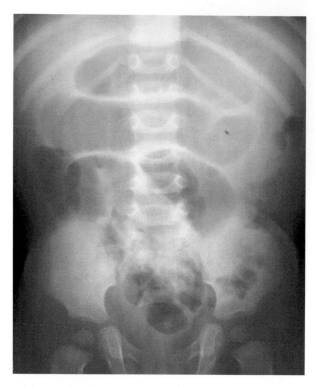

**Fig. 5.2**   Intussusception. Small bowel distension and absence of caecal shadow.

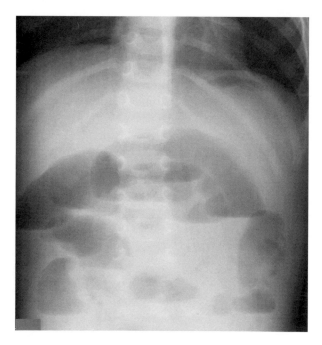

**Fig. 5.3**   Intussusception. Erect position showing fluid levels.

and, therefore, an erect chest X-ray should be undertaken to exclude perforation prior to such intervention[10].

## Appendicitis

Appendicitis can occur at any age and is the most common cause of acute abdominal symptoms in children over 5 years of age[6,12]. In children younger than 5 years of age the classic clinical symptoms of right lower quadrant pain, leukocytosis and vomiting are found in only 50% of patients and careful clinical assessment is required. Appendicitis is essentially a clinical diagnosis and imaging is only required in equivocal cases. In these cases, ultrasound is the imaging modality of choice[5] and a gentle, graded compression technique may demonstrate a thick-walled inflammatory appendix mass in the right iliac fossa.

## Hernia

Hernias are usually congenital muscular defects through which bowel and other abdominal organs may prolapse into a body cavity in which they are not normally located[5] (Box 5.1).

## Gastroesophageal reflux

Gastroesophageal reflux is common in infants up to 8 weeks of age because of functional immaturity and abnormal tone of the lower oesophageal sphincter[4]. The most common clinical symptom is non-bilious vomiting but other signs include failure to thrive and rectal bleeding in infants and young children, while older children may present with heartburn and dysphagia[11]. The barium meal examination is a relatively insensitive method of detecting oesophageal reflux because of the short period of time over which the patient is examined. The current diagnostic investigation of choice is 24-hour pH probe monitoring[11].

## Meckel's diverticulum

A Meckel's diverticulum is a developmental abnormality resulting in a small pouch on the wall of the lower part of the ileum. The condition is relatively common and generally asymptomatic. However, inflammation of the diverticulum (diverticulitis) may cause painless rectal bleeding, intestinal obstruction and localised abdominal pain mimicking appendicitis[6]. The peak incidence of symptomatic cases is around 2 years of age. Radiological diagnosis of Meckel's diverticulum is difficult unless haemorrhage occurs. Scintigraphy is the imaging modality of choice[11].

## Inflammatory bowel disease

Inflammatory bowel disease is a collective term for a range of inflammatory conditions including ulcerative colitis and Crohn's disease (regional ileitis) (Fig. 5.5).

**Box 5.1**   Common sites of herniation.

*Diaphragmatic hernia*
*Acquired:*   Herniation of an abdominal organ into the thoracic cavity. The most common type, hiatus hernia, involves the stomach passing through the oesophageal opening in the diaphragm.

*Congenital:*   The most common is the Bochdalek hernia, a postero-lateral defect more common on the left than the right. The anterior, Morgagni type defect is less common and usually smaller (Fig. 5.4).

*Umbilical hernia*
Results from the incomplete closure of the fascia of the umbilical ring and is more common in premature and black infants[6]. An umbilical hernia usually presents during the neonatal period as a bulge at the navel[13], and many resolve spontaneously, although strangulation of the hernia remains a risk with conservative management. Diagnosis is based on clinical examination and imaging is not required unless the clinical diagnosis is equivocal or the exact contents of the hernia need to be determined preoperatively.

*Inguinal hernia*
More common in males than females, the inguinal hernia is a prolapse of the bowel through the inguinal ring. The condition may be asymptomatic although compression of other organs may produce associated symptoms. Conservative management can lead to intestinal obstruction if the lesion becomes swollen and fixed (incarcerated) or if the blood supply is compromised (strangulation) causing pain and gangrene[13]. A sliding hernia can result in bowel wall irritation and functional obstruction[13].

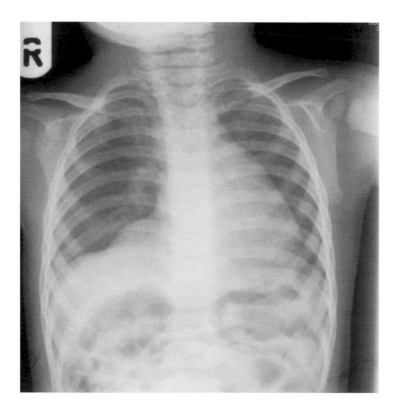

**Fig. 5.4**   Morgagni herniation. Herniation of the liver through the diaphragm (right cardiophrenic angle).

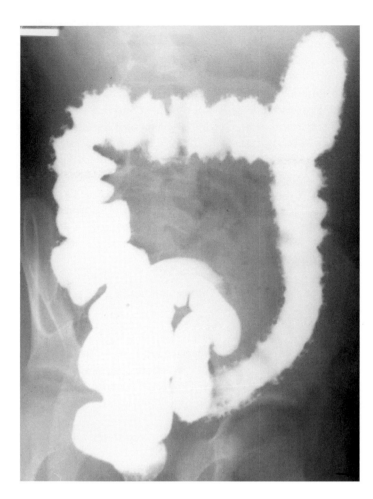

**Fig. 5.5**   Colitis. Evidence of extensive ulceration.

Approximately 25% of all cases of inflammatory bowel disease first manifest during childhood and these form the most common chronic gastrointestinal illnesses in children and adolescents[11]. Presenting signs include weight loss and diarrhoea. Radiographic appearances during gastrointestinal contrast examinations tend to be similar to those undertaken in adults. However, ultrasound has a greater role to play in the investigation of inflammatory bowel disease in children as the paediatric bowel wall may be technically easier to visualise than in adults[11].

## Swallowed foreign body

Most ingested foreign bodies will pass unimpeded through the gastrointestinal tract and plain film radiography is not routinely indicated unless the swallowed object is sharp or potentially poisonous (e.g. a safety pin or a watch battery), or if there is clinical concern that the object has become lodged in the abdomen[9,10].

The most likely sites for foreign bodies to become impacted are the pharynx, mid-oesophagus, where the left main bronchus crosses anteriorly, and at the gastroesophageal junction. While objects passing through these sites are likely to have an uneventful transit through the rest of the gastrointestinal tract, long thin foreign bodies may lodge in the duodenal loop or terminal ileum[10]. If clinical concern exists for an infant an antero-posterior projection of the chest and upper abdomen should be performed with the patient in the supine position and the head turned laterally. The radiograph should be collimated to include the pharynx superiorly and the iliac crests inferiorly thereby excluding the gonads from the primary beam. For the older child, separate radiographic examinations of the chest (including the upper pharyngeal region) and abdomen may be requested.

If a foreign body is identified in the neck or thorax then a lateral projection of this region should be undertaken to verify the object's position within the pharynx or oesophagus and to exclude inhalation (Fig. 5.6).

# Genitourinary system pathology

## Urinary tract infection

Urinary tract infections are a common, important paediatric problem and are a significant cause of childhood morbidity. Urinary tract infections occur more commonly in females than males and early investigation of a proven bacterial infection is essential in order to prevent parenchymal scarring and progressive renal failure.

Clinical symptoms of urinary tract infection vary with patient age and may be non-specific in children under 6 years of age (Table 5.1).

All proven urinary tract infections require diagnostic imaging to assess the extent of renal damage and to diagnose vesicoureteric reflux. Ultrasound may be useful as the initial imaging examination to demonstrate cortical scarring and pelvi-caliceal dilatation. However, micturating cystourethrography and scintigraphy are considered the gold standard investigations for reflux and scarring, respectively.

**Table 5.1**  Symptoms of urinary tract infection (UTI).

| Age | Symptoms |
| --- | --- |
| 1 month to 2 years | Failure to thrive<br>Feeding problems<br>Diarrhoea<br>Unexplained fever<br>UTI in this age group can also masquerade as gastrointestinal colic. |
| 2–6 years | Non-specific symptoms as above<br>  or<br>Classic urinary tract infection symptoms of urgency, dysuria, frequency and abdominal pain. |
| 6–18 years | Classic symptoms of urgency, dysuria, frequency and abdominal pain. |

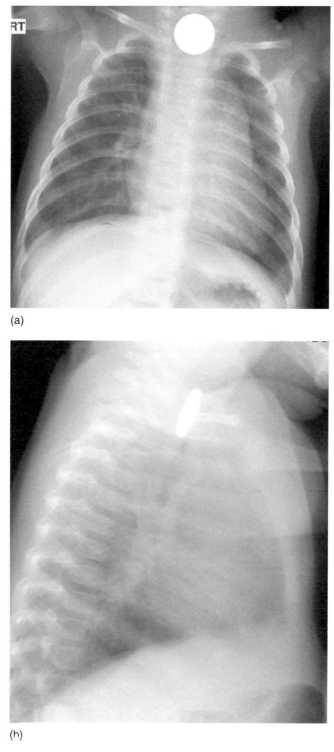

(a)

(h)

**Fig. 5.6** (a) Coin identified within the neck (antero-posterior projection). (b) Coin position confirmed within oesophagus (lateral projection).

Isolated renal calculi are extremely rare in children and plain film radiography is only appropriate as a control image prior to contrast examinations.

## Vesicoureteric reflux

Abnormal retrograde flow of urine from the bladder into the ureter and renal collecting system is termed vesicoureteric reflux. Reflux may occur as a result of a congenital abnormality at the vesicoureteric junction or may be associated with a neurogenic bladder or a partial bladder outlet obstruction. Reflux is significant because it predisposes the whole of the urinary tract to ascending infection. Chronic or recurrent inflammation of the kidney (pyelonephritis) can lead to renal cortical scarring with increased risk of hypertension and renal failure in later life.

## Hydronephrosis

Hydronephrosis is the dilation of the renal pelvi-caliceal collecting system proximal to an obstructing lesion (Fig. 5.7) and is common in neonates presenting

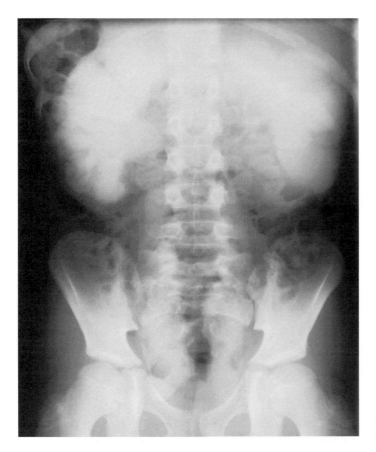

**Fig. 5.7**  Hydronephrosis. Dilation of the collecting system above an obstruction.

with an abdominal mass[6]. A pelvi-ureteric junction obstruction is the commonest cause of hydronephrosis and may result from intrinsic stenosis, functional obstruction or compression of the pelvi-ureteric junction by an aberrant artery or fibrous band.

Unilateral or bilateral hydronephrosis can be seen in the presence of a uterocele at the vesicoureteric junction and will also be associated with dilatation of the ureter(s). Simple renal dilatation can occur without obstruction in conditions such as vesicoureteric reflux and in such cases may be a transient phenomenon.

## Posterior urethral valves

Posterior urethral valves are the commonest cause of lower urinary tract obstruction in boys and result from mucosal folds that obstruct the urethra and cause bladder outlet obstruction. The diagnosis is often made prenatally with ultrasound showing a dilated fetal urinary system and reduced amniotic fluid volume. Posterior urethral valves may be detected in the postnatal period following clinical examination of a healthy neonate with a distended bladder and poor urinary stream. Occasionally the condition presents with overflow incontinence or urinary tract infection in later childhood. Micturating cystourethrography in these cases will demonstrate bilateral obstructive hydronephrosis which may also be associated with vesicoureteric reflux[7].

## Haematuria

Blood in the urine of a child is a non-specific indicator of genitourinary disease and, in the absence of recent surgery or trauma, is usually the result of bacterial infection. Rarely, haematuria may occur as a result of a urinary tract calculus or neoplasm and in these circumstances abdominal ultrasound or contrast urography is indicated.

## Renal agenesis

Absence of one or both kidneys is usually diagnosed during routine antenatal ultrasound screening. Bilateral renal agenesis is incompatible with life and an affected child will succumb early in the neonatal period. Unilateral renal agenesis will cause compensatory hypertrophy of the contra-lateral kidney and the child may have normal, or only minimally reduced, overall renal function[14].

There is a spectrum of congenital variations in renal anatomy that result from the abnormal migration of the kidneys from the pelvis to the upper abdomen during embryonic life. Common variants include the abnormal location of one or both kidneys (ectopic kidney) and crossed renal ectopia. The ectopic kidney will usually be located at the pelvic brim (Fig. 5.8) whereas crossed renal ectopia will result in both kidneys being located on the same side. Occasionally, bilateral kidneys are joined at the upper or lower poles creating a 'horseshoe' kidney (Fig. 5.9) or alternatively duplication or partial duplication of the renal pelvis

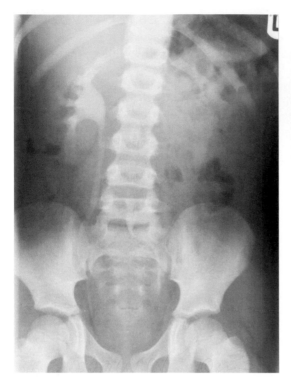

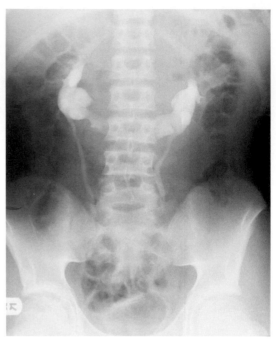

**Fig. 5.9**   Horseshoe kidney. The lower poles are joined. Fusion of the lower poles is more typical than joining at the upper poles.

**Fig. 5.8**   Ectopic kidney. The left kidney is located over the sacrum.

and ureter may occur (duplex kidney). All of these anomalies may be demonstrated using ultrasound or contrast urography.

### Chronic renal failure

Chronic renal failure occurs when causative abnormalities are not detected early enough to allow intervention. The causative mechanisms in children are closely related to the age of the child at the time renal failure manifests. Below the age of 5 years, congenital obstructive malformations and hereditary renal dysplasias are the most common cause whereas in children over the age of 5 years, acquired disease resulting in progressive renal scarring is more likely[6].

### Undescended testes (cryptorchidism)

Undescended testes are present in 0.7% of males above 1 year of age although the incidence is greater at birth. Spontaneous testicular descent may occur during the first year of life but above this age, poor testicular development and atrophy will occur. Accurate diagnosis of the condition is important as malignant change in undescended testes has been reported in 20–44% of cases, usually in the third and fourth decades of life[6]. Ultrasound will often demonstrate an abdominal

testis in the inguinal canal although in a significant number of cases undescended testes may be associated with other genitourinary tract anomalies and
evaluation of the whole genitourinary system is prudent.

### Abdominal mass

In children under 4 years of age, an abdominal mass is likely to involve the renal
system and is most commonly due to hydronephrosis[4,15], although abdominal
malignancies should be actively excluded. Ultrasound is the imaging modality
of choice and will readily allow identification of the affected organs and assessment of any mass effect or invasion of adjacent structures[9,10,15]. The most common
paediatric abdominal malignancies are neuroblastoma (adrenal), Wilms' tumour
(kidney), hepatoblastoma and hepatocellular carcinoma (liver), rhabdomyosar-
coma (skeletal muscle) and lymphoma.

### Nephroblastoma (Wilms' tumour)

Nephroblastoma, or Wilms' tumour, is a malignant tumour of the renal
parenchyma and is the most common solid abdominal tumour in childhood.
It usually manifests as a firm, painless upper abdominal mass and bilateral
involvement is noted in 5–10% of patients[11]. Approximately 90% of Wilms'
tumours are diagnosed before the age of 7 years[12]. A Wilms' tumour may be
apparent as an upper abdominal soft tissue mass on plain films (Fig. 5.10), but
ultrasound will localise the mass to the kidney and allow assessment of local
spread. Ultrasound is also useful as a non-invasive examination for long-
term follow-up. Computed tomography may be required for comprehensive tumour staging and with prompt surgical resection and neo-adjuvant
chemotherapy, the prognosis for nephroblastoma is good with a greater than 90%
5-year survival rate.

# Signs and symptoms of abdominal pathology

### Abdominal pain

Acute abdominal pain commonly signifies gastroenteritis in young children[7] but
may also be indicative of trauma, intussusception, incarcerated hernia, renal tract
infection, volvulus and malrotation. In older children (2–5 years) systemic conditions such as sickle cell anaemia or chest pathology (e.g. lower lobe pneumonia) may also present with abdominal pain, while in children aged 5 years
or over a diagnosis of appendicitis should be given primary consideration[6].
Imaging in cases of acute abdominal pain is dependent upon the clinical symptoms, suspected clinical diagnosis and the age of the child. Plain film radiography of the chest and abdomen or abdominal and pelvic ultrasound may both be
considered as first-line imaging investigations[10] and the imaging protocols are
likely and to be dependent upon modality availability and local expertise.

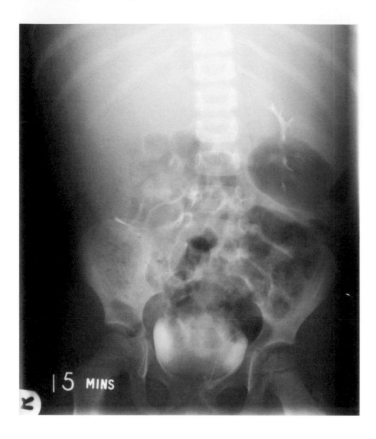

**Fig. 5.10**  Nephroblastoma. Large right renal mass. Displacement of the right renal collecting system.

## Vomiting

Vomiting is an extremely common non-specific sign of abdominal pathology. However, the character of the vomitus and the age of the child can assist in the provision of a differential diagnosis (Table 5.2). Imaging is not routinely indicated in cases of isolated childhood vomiting, but where the vomiting is projectile and sustained, hypertrophic pyloric stenosis should be suspected and ultrasound performed[9].

**Table 5.2**  Differential diagnosis for vomiting in childhood[12].

| Age | Non-bilious vomit | Bilious vomit |
| --- | --- | --- |
| Birth–2 months | Gastroesophageal reflux<br>Pyloric stenosis | Midgut volvulus<br>Small bowel obstruction<br>Bowel atresia<br>Hirschprung's disease |
| 2 months–2 years | Rarely an organic cause | Small bowel obstruction<br>Intussusception<br>Midgut volvulus |
| Over 2 years | Most causes not related to gastrointestinal tract abnormality | |

**Table 5.3**  Causes of gastrointestinal bleeding[16].

| Age | Cause of bleeding |
| --- | --- |
| Neonate | Necrotising enterocolitis<br>Infectious colitis |
| Infant | Stress ulcer<br>Meckel's diverticulum<br>Intussusception |
| Child | Polyp<br>Inflammatory bowel disease |

## Gastrointestinal bleeding

Causes of intestinal bleeding are listed in Table 5.3. Scintigraphy is the imaging modality of choice to locate the source of an intestinal bleed. However endoscopy, in preference to barium studies, and ultrasound may demonstrate changes associated with inflammatory bowel disease or intussusception[9].

## Constipation

Abdominal radiography will show extensive faecal material as a normal feature in many children and therefore imaging is not helpful in the diagnosis or management of constipation and should not be performed routinely[9].

## Chronic diarrhoea

Chronic diarrhoea is a non-specific sign of abdominal pathology. Clinical diagnosis relies heavily on patient medical history and the pathological assessment of stool specimens. Barium examinations, if undertaken, may show signs of inflammatory bowel disease. However, for many patients presenting with diarrhoea as a result of a small bowel mucosal disorder, only a non-specific malabsorption pattern (thickened mucosal folds, bowel wall oedema, barium flocculation) will be seen[6] and, in these cases, more invasive diagnostic investigations (e.g. jejunoscopy) should be considered.

## Gastric dilatation

An over-distended gas-filled stomach can result from air swallowing during crying and is therefore a common finding on plain film radiographs of young infants and children. Only when little or no air is seen in the bowel distal to a distended stomach should concerns be raised and gastric outlet obstruction considered[4].

# Radiographic technique for the abdomen

## Plain film abdominal radiography

There is no specific preparation for radiography of the paediatric abdomen. However, general preparation such as providing a procedural explanation will be necessary in order to gain the child's confidence and co-operation, and such an explanation should be modified to accommodate the child's level of under-standing. It is not always necessary to undress a child fully for plain film radi-ography of the abdomen but, when required, an appropriately sized examination gown should be provided. It is often possible to move clothes away from the area of interest without removing them entirely and this helps to maintain the dignity of the child. It should be remembered that even relatively young chil-dren are aware of their own sexuality and will feel uncomfortable with their clothes removed in the presence of strangers. In male children, underpants can be left on and lowered to the level of the symphysis pubis while still covering the genitalia. Lowering the underpants in this way also ensures that the testicles are displaced from the region of interest and are not within the primary beam (Fig. 5.11).

The antero-posterior projection of the abdomen, with the patient in the supine position, is the initial projection of choice for paediatric abdominal referrals. Additional antero-posterior projections with the patient erect or lying in the lateral decubitus position are occasionally necessary, but these projections should not be performed routinely. If a decubitus projection is required to demonstrate 'free air' within the abdomen then the left lateral decubitus is preferable to the

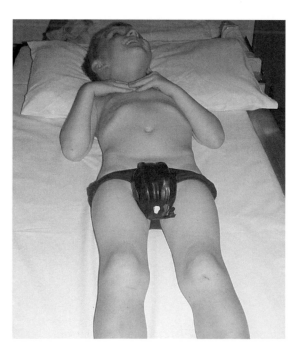

**Fig. 5.11** Gonad protection for a male patient. The capsule covers the gonads but does not obscure the lower abdomen.

right to prevent any 'free air' being confused with gas in the stomach. In addition, if perforation is suspected then an erect chest projection should also be undertaken as small amounts of free air under the diaphragm are easier to identify on images produced using typical chest exposure factors.

### Supine abdomen

Radiographic positioning for paediatric abdominal radiography is not significantly different to adult radiography of the abdomen although *maintaining* the correct position often requires the creative use of distraction and immobilisation techniques (Fig. 5.12). Figure 5.13 illustrates a child being positioned for an antero-posterior projection of the abdomen in the supine position. To avoid rotation and movement prior to, or during, exposure the child's hands are positioned near to their shoulders and held by the accompanying adult. A Bucky binder or sand bags may be applied over the child's legs to aid immobilisation. Older children do not usually require the use of such immobilisation techniques as they are less inquisitive and more inclined to co-operate with the radiographer.

The paediatric abdomen is frequently as wide as it is long so care must be taken with choice of film size and collimation. A common radiographic error is to collimate within the lateral margins of the abdomen and this often prevents evaluation of the whole of the abdomen since the lateral edges of some organs will be excluded (Fig. 5.14).

Radiographic exposure should be made on arrested respiration following expiration. In children too young to co-operate by holding their breath, the

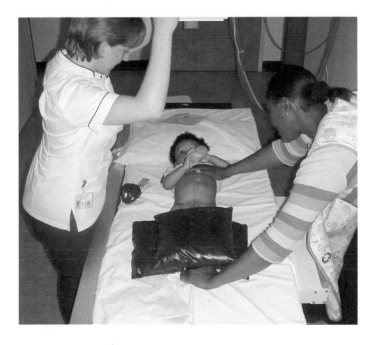

**Fig. 5.12** The child is enjoying a drink which is helping to pacify him during the preparation for an abdominal x-ray.

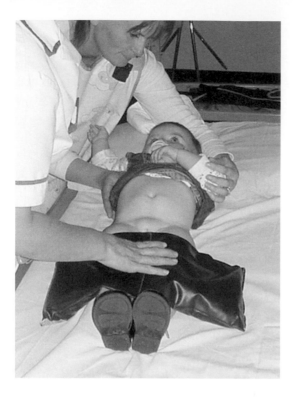

**Fig. 5.13** The guardian is close to the child's head to offer emotional support whilst holding the shoulders to prevent rotation.

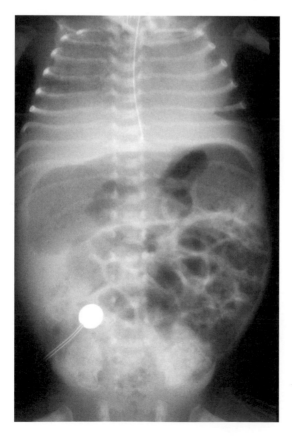

**Fig. 5.14** The properitoneal fat lines should be included on the radiograph. If they are excluded from the radiograph there is a possibility that some of the abdominal contents will be excluded.

radiographer must observe the natural rise and fall of the abdomen during spontaneous respiration, and make the exposure accordingly.

It is not appropriate to define a specific anatomical centring point for paediatric abdominal radiography because of the varying relative abdominal and pelvic proportions during normal growth. Instead, to ensure that the whole of the abdomen is included on the radiographic image, the lower border of an appropriately sized cassette should be positioned to include the symphysis pubis inferiorly and the central ray directed to the middle of the cassette through the median sagittal plane.

### Erect abdomen

Figure 5.15 illustrates an antero-posterior projection of the abdomen with the patient positioned erect using a horizontal central ray. A horizontal central ray is required to demonstrate an air–fluid interface that may be of value in the investigation of intestinal obstruction or perforation. However, the erect abdomen should not be undertaken routinely in the investigation of these conditions.

### Lateral decubitus

Figure 5.16 illustrates a postero-anterior projection with the patient in the left lateral decubitus position. A postero-anterior projection is advocated in

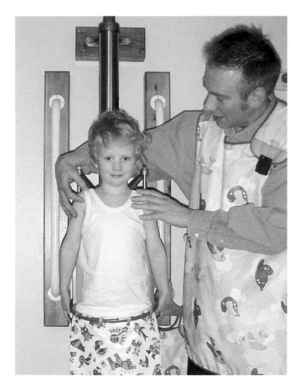

**Fig. 5.15** Erect abdomen. A guardian provides close support whilst excluded from the primary beam. A waist apron provides gonad protection. Support at the shoulders ensures that there is no rotation.

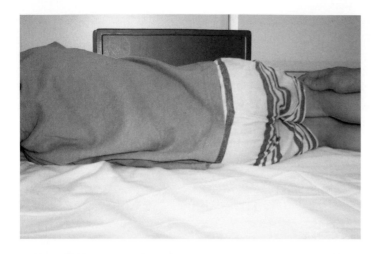

**Fig. 5.16**  A postero-anterior projection with the patient in the left lateral decubitus position. The mattress ensures the lower flank is above the bottom of the cassette and will be included on the film which is positioned on the table top and supported with pads.

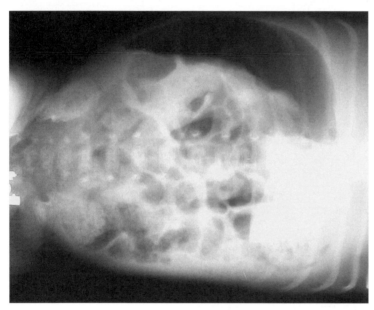

**Fig. 5.17**  An antero-posterior projection of the abdomen with the patient lying in the lateral decubitus position and demonstrating free abdominal air.

preference to the antero-posterior projection in order to reduce the dose to radiosensitive organs that lie anteriorly within the body.

An advantage of the lateral decubitus position, when compared to the erect projection taken with the child sitting, is that the patient's thighs are positioned so as not to obscure the lower abdominal region. The lateral decubitus position is also easier to achieve and more comfortable to maintain when imaging very sick children (Fig. 5.17).

### Lateral abdomen

In cases of suspected bowel perforation, moving the patient from the supine position may not be recommended or possible, and in such circumstances a lateral projection of the abdomen with the patient supine may be necessary (Fig. 5.18). This projection will demonstrate free air as a small triangle of gas anterior to the haustral folds along the anterior abdominal wall (Fig. 5.19). However, accurate recognition of free air in the peritoneal cavity may be hindered if the radiograph is over-exposed for this region and a reduction in overall exposure factors or use of a wedge filter should be employed to modify the standard local lateral abdominal exposure factors.

### Exposure factors and radiation protection

Table 5.4 outlines typical exposure factor combinations for abdominal radiography across a range of paediatric ages. These examples assume that additional filtration has been added to the x-ray tube as recommended by the European Guidelines on Quality Criteria for Diagnostic Radiographic Images in

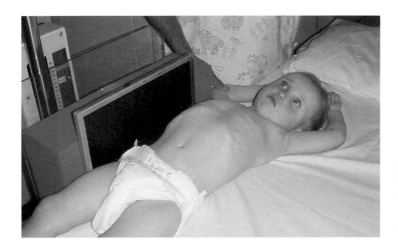

**Fig. 5.18** A child positioned for the lateral abdomen in the supine decubitus position. The arms are raised above the head and a guardian is positioned to comfort the child.

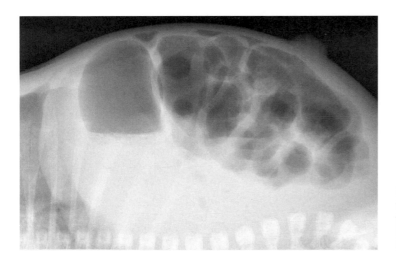

**Fig. 5.19** A lateral projection of the abdomen with the patient in the supine decubitus position. Free gas is visible against the anterior abdominal wall.

**Table 5.4**  Exposure factors – guidelines for abdominal radiography.

| Age (years) | Focal spot | Kilovoltage (kV) | mAs (exposure time less than 0.02s) | FFD[a] (cm) | Relative screen/ film speed | Grid | AEC[b] |
|---|---|---|---|---|---|---|---|
| <1 | Fine | 60 | 2 | 100–115 | 400 | No | No |
| 1–4 | Fine | 75 | 4 | 100–115 | 400 | Yes/No (dependent upon size) | No |
| 4+ | Broad (used to keep exposure time down) | 75 | AEC | 100–115 | 400 | Yes | Yes |

[a] Focus-to-film distance.
[b] Automatic exposure control.

Paediatrics[17]. Since there is a natural variation in the size and shape of children of the same age, the examining radiographer will need to modify any standard or guideline exposure factors according to the individual patient, clinical presentation and the imaging equipment used.

The use of an automatic exposure control (AEC) requires careful consideration by the examining radiographer and a convincing case can be made against their use with small children. The relatively small size of the child compared to the ionisation chamber often makes it difficult to position and maintain the dominant abdominal area over the selected chamber and can result in suboptimal exposure of the radiograph. Care must also be taken with equipment where AEC operation is dependent upon the use of a grid as this will automatically necessitate an increase in exposure factors and, therefore, patient dose without an obvious significant increase in the resultant image quality.

## Radiographic assessment criteria

The radiograph must satisfy specific criteria in terms of patient position and exposure. When correctly positioned the resultant image should clearly demonstrate the ischial tuberosities, diaphragm and lateral abdominal walls. The spine should be positioned centrally and appear symmetrical in the midline with no evidence of rotation. A correctly exposed image will allow soft tissue structures (such as the psoas muscle), properitoneal fat stripes, and renal and hepatic outlines, to be visualised. A radiograph of the abdomen should demonstrate evidence of primary beam collimation to within all four edges of the image, although additional collimation can be applied limiting the primary beam to that portion of the abdomen containing the renal tract (upper poles of the kidneys down to the proximal urethra) when radiography is being undertaken specifically for renal tract pathology.

# Fluoroscopic examinations

To ensure that the maximum diagnostic information is obtained with the minimum radiation dose, all paediatric fluoroscopic examinations should be recorded on video tape. In addition, automatic brightness controls should not be used and grids should be removed prior to the examination of very small children. The introduction of a contrast agent will increase the subject contrast and facilitate the use of a high kilovoltage (kV) technique (e.g. 75 kVp for infants, 90 kVp for 5 year-olds). Dual field image intensifiers allow magnification of the fluoroscopic image with potentially improved spatial and contrast resolution and this is often useful when imaging small babies. However, this facility should be used prudently as possible associations with increased patient dose have been documented[18].

The primary beam should be tightly collimated to the area of interest and the number of radiographic images kept to the minimum necessary to achieve an accurate diagnosis. Ideally, images should be recorded from the output of the image intensifier either digitally or using 100 mm cut film or thermal imagers. A dose-area product (DAP) meter should be attached to the fluoroscopy X-ray tube and the output readings documented to allow patient dose calculations to be undertaken. The DAP readings should also be subject to regular audit to identify erroneous readings, quality assurance problems and poor fluoroscopic technique. If an under-couch fluoroscopy unit is used, care must be taken to avoid injuring the child with the explorator and the vertical locking device should be employed at an acceptable examination height to prevent unintentional compression of the child.

# Gastrointestinal tract examinations

## Barium swallow and meal

Barium swallow and meal examinations are used to diagnose, or exclude, gastroesophageal reflux and congenital abnormalities of the upper gastrointestinal tract (e.g. malrotation). Physical preparation of the patient is age dependent:

*Barium meal and swallow: patient preparation*

| | |
|---|---|
| 0–2 years | Nil by mouth 3 hours prior to examination. |
| Over 2 years | Nil by mouth 6 hours prior to examination and high residue diet avoided. |

For infants and young children a single contrast swallow and meal technique is used. Iso-osmolar water-soluble contrast media are the contrast agents of choice for initial examination of the *neonatal* gastrointestinal tract as they are quickly absorbed and are less hazardous if they enter the peritoneal cavity or bronchial tree[19]. These agents should also be used in older children whenever perforation is suspected or inhalation likely, although they are unpalatable even when flavoured. Beyond the neonatal period, fruit-flavoured barium sulphate preparations are normally used and are reasonably well tolerated by the majority of children.

The technique for examination of the paediatric upper gastrointestinal tract is similar to that for adults. With the child lying on their right side, dilute barium sulphate (i.e. 50% w/v) is administered orally from a feeding bottle or through a straw from a cup held by the guardian. If a feeding bottle is used, the teat must have relatively large holes to allow the barium suspension to pass through. Lateral spot images of the lower pharynx and oesophagus are taken in this position as the contrast agent passes down the oesophagus.

While the child maintains this lateral position, the stomach and duodenum are observed and a lateral image taken of the gastric outlet and second part of the duodenum. The child is then rolled to demonstrate different parts of the stomach and duodenal loop (Fig. 5.20). These projections must be taken early in the examination as a contrast-filled stomach and small bowel will eventually obscure the duodenal–jejunal flexure[10]. Visualisation of the duodenal–jejunal flexure is important as, in cases of malrotation, it is commonly displaced inferiorly and to the right[13]. If necessary a small infant may be picked up and fed by their guardian at this point before being returned to the examination table; images of the lower oesophagus and stomach are then taken with the child in the supine position.

If reflux is suspected then it may be stimulated by gently rolling the patient from side to side or applying abdominal pressure while the patient sips a non-barium drink.

A double-contrast upper gastrointestinal examination technique is possible with older children and the technique is similar to that adopted with adult patients. Again demonstration of the duodenal–jejunal flexure position is important.

## Barium follow-through

A barium follow-through examination is indicated for conditions such as failure to thrive, Crohn's disease, partial obstruction associated with malrotation, diarrhoea and chronic vomiting. The patient is prepared as for the barium meal examination although for older children/adolescents a slightly longer 'nil by mouth' period and mild laxatives may be necessary. It is important that patients and guardians are aware of the examination procedure and its likely length prior to attending the imaging department, although the latter is somewhat indeterminate and patient specific.

A limited barium meal is often appropriate prior to a follow-through examination to assess gastric emptying and demonstrate the duodenal–jejunal flexure.

The follow-through examination involves taking well-collimated postero-anterior images, with the patient in the prone position, at time intervals specified by the supervising radiologist. The exact number and timing of exposures will be dependent on the patient's condition and clinical history. Prone positioning allows natural compression of the bowel, separates the bowel loops and reduces radiation dose to sensitive structures. However, if immobilised prone

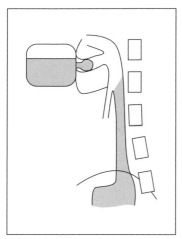

**Image 1**
Patient in right lateral decubitus position. Oesophagus visualised.

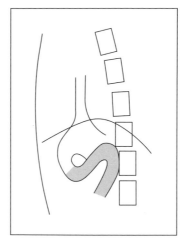

**Image 2**
Patient in right lateral decubitus position. Gastric outlet and second part of duodenum visualised.

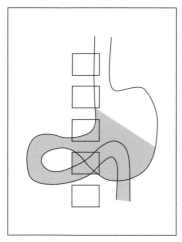

**Image 3**
Gastric antrum and first and second part of duodenum visualised.

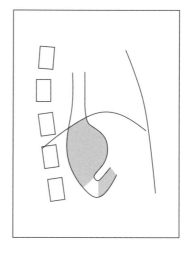

**Image 4**
Patient in left lateral decubitus position. Fundus and third part of duodenum visualised.

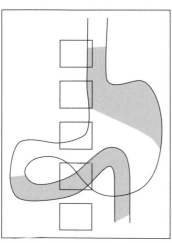

**Image 5**
Duodenal–jejunal flexure seen through gas-filled antrum. There must be no rotation of the patient for the projection.

**Fig. 5.20** Early images acquired during a barium meal.

positioning is not possible, images may be taken with the patient in the supine position. Periodic fluoroscopy is also required during the procedure to demonstrate areas of overlying bowel loops and is particularly useful for examining the terminal ileum after contrast has passed through into the caecum.

### Small bowel enema

Visualisation of the small bowel can be achieved with a modified follow-through examination – the small bowel enema. This examination allows more rapid and complete visualisation of the small bowel but does not examine the oesophagus, stomach or duodenum. The patient is fasted for 12 hours prior to examination, although they may take small sips of clear fluids. Any antispasmodic drugs should be withheld for 24 hours prior to examination. Mild laxatives may be required for older children.

If not already *in situ*, a nasogastric tube is passed and advanced into the fourth part of the duodenum. The position of the tube is checked under fluoroscopic control prior to the administration of contrast. Insertion of the tube often requires patient sedation. Dilute barium sulphate is administered rapidly through the nasogastric tube and monitored under fluoroscopic control. Localised fluoroscopic and full-length images are taken as required to demonstrate the anatomy of the small bowel. During the withdrawal of the nasogastric tube, the contrast agent is aspirated to decrease the risk of inhalation[20]. When examining very young infants, water-soluble contrast agents should be used in preference to barium suspensions.

The small bowel enema examination is contraindicated if the child is unwilling or unable to co-operate, as compliance is essential for a successful study. The patient should refrain from eating or drinking for 4 hours post-examination or until the effects of the sedation have worn off and the guardian should be warned that the child may subsequently have diarrhoea.

### Barium enema

There is no specific physical preparation for the barium enema examination for babies less than 1 year old, patients suffering from Hirschprung's disease or those with active colitis. For all other patients, the colon should be cleared of faecal matter and this can be achieved with a low residue diet and administration of a mild laxative for up to 48 hours prior to the examination. It is important that young children are well hydrated and encouraged to drink plenty of fluids before and after the examination. Children over the age of 5 years may be fasted for 12 hours prior to the examination but should be given the earliest available morning appointment to minimise inconvenience and distress.

The barium enema examination is indicated for any pathology that may result in large bowel obstruction (e.g. intussusception, Hirschprung's disease, neoplasm) or when inflammatory bowel disease is suspected. A low osmolar iodine-based contrast agent should be used in preference to a barium preparation when examining neonates and young infants or when bowel perforation is suspected.

In contrast, if a meconium ileus is suspected then a high osmolar iodine-based contrast agent may be used as it has a hydroscopic effect and can be therapeutic, causing softening of the meconium and relieving the obstruction. However, if a high osmolar contrast agent is used then care should be taken to avoid dehydration of the neonate.

The child's age and suspected pathology influence the choice of radiographic technique employed. When examining very young children, a single-contrast examination will provide a diagnosis in the majority of cases whereas in the examination of older children, or where inflammatory bowel disease is suspected, a double-contrast technique should be used.

In a single-contrast examination, the patient should lie on their left side with their hips and knees flexed. A soft rubber catheter is gently inserted into the rectum and taped into position. The patient maintains the lateral position while a 30–100g/100ml suspension of barium sulphate[10], warmed to body temperature, is introduced slowly under gravitational force. Progress of the contrast agent through the bowel is monitored fluoroscopically and images taken to demonstrate large bowel anatomy. Routine images might include a lateral projection of the rectum, right and left posterior oblique projections for the splenic and hepatic flexures and an antero-posterior projection to demonstrate the caecum and terminal ileum.

A double-contrast technique is similar to the above except that a higher concentration barium sulphate suspension, 60–120g/100ml, is used and the technique also includes air insufflation. Antero-posterior projections in the prone position, with 45° caudal angulation of the central ray to show the sigmoid colon, and lateral decubitus projections, may be required for a complete study, but are not routinely taken.

Air enemas may also be used to reduce intussusception. In these cases, anti-spasmodic agents may be given prior to examination to relax the bowel after which air at a pressure not exceeding 80mmHg is insufflated over 3 minutes. The child should be rested for 3 minutes before repeating this procedure. At no time should the pressure exceed 120mmHg[10] and a maximum of three attempts should be made. In a successful examination, fluoroscopy will demonstrate air bubbling through the site of the intussusception. Surgical reduction may be required if the image-guided reduction attempt fails, and surgical staff should be made aware of the procedure in case of a surgical emergency. Contraindications to the air enema are suspected perforation or peritonitis.

# Renal tract examinations

## Intravenous urography

Ultrasound is the initial imaging examination of choice for renal tract pathology in the child and intravenous urography (IVU) is required only when less invasive procedures have failed to provide adequate diagnostic information.

Prior to administration of a contrast agent, the child should be weighed and the dose calculated in accordance with the manufacturer's instructions on volume and concentration in terms of iodine content per kilogram of body weight. A topical local anaesthetic should be applied to several potential injection sites at least 1 hour prior to radiographic examination to facilitate intravenous puncture or, alternatively, the contrast agent may be administered through an existing intravenous line where one is already *in situ*.

It is standard practice to starve the patient for 4 hours prior to the administration of a contrast agent in order to ensure that the stomach is empty. However, it is important that patients, particularly children, remain well hydrated and clear fluids should not be restricted. Flexibility in examination appointment times, particularly for infants and young children, will be necessary so that the examination can be timed for when the stomach is likely to be empty (i.e. timed to coincide with a milk feed). Following contrast agent injection, infants may be bottle-fed to help pacify them. The fluid-filled stomach will effectively form a radiographic 'window' facilitating the visualisation of the renal area.

Each IVU examination should be tailored to the individual patient and directed to answer a specific clinical question[13] thereby ensuring that the number of radiographic images taken is kept to a minimum. Ideally, the renal tract should be visualised free from overlying bowel gas and faeces, and the use of ureteric compression and oblique projections may be required to achieve this. Oral carbonated drinks can be used in older children to distend the stomach and provide a gaseous 'window' through which the kidneys may be visualised; the antero-posterior projection with the patient supine demonstrating the left kidney while a right posterior oblique will demonstrate the right kidney. Alternatively, the kidneys may be visualised by an antero-posterior projection with the patient supine and 35° caudal angulation centred to the xiphisternum. This will project any bowel gas below the renal outlines.

## Micturating cystourethrography

Micturating cystourethrography (MCU) is the definitive method of assessing the lower urinary tract[13]. It is particularly valuable for the assessment of male urethral pathology (e.g. posterior urethral valves and urethral strictures) and for demonstrating vesicoureteric reflux, a common cause of recurrent urinary tract infection.

This examination requires a small catheter to be inserted into the bladder via the urethra and although this procedure is performed under strict asepsis, it is still associated with a finite risk of urinary tract infection. As a result, prophylactic antibiotic cover may be prescribed prior to the examination or post-examination if warranted by the diagnostic outcome (e.g. reflux is demonstrated). Micturating cystourethrography is contraindicated in cases of proven current infection or where a documented infection has occurred during the 4-week period prior to the examination.

It is important that a clear and honest explanation of the procedure is given to the child and their guardian prior to entering the imaging room and written informed consent must be obtained. In departments where micturating cystourethrography is commonly performed, a special doll with interchangeable genitalia may be used to demonstrate the catheterisation technique in order to reduce anxiety and maximise co-operation. Micturating cystourethrography will invariably involve soiling the child's clothing and therefore the child should be changed into a paediatric hospital gown or, in the case of very young children, hospital-owned vest and top. Alternatively the patient may prefer to wear their own, familiar clothes and should be instructed to bring a change of suitable clothing with them.

The child lies supine on the examination table and the guardian, wearing an appropriate protective apron, is positioned near the child's head where they can offer emotional support and encouragement. The child's legs are abducted and flexed at the hips and knees and the soles of the feet are brought together – the 'frog lateral' position. Using a strict aseptic technique, the penis or perineum is cleaned with an antiseptic solution. A 4–8 French sized catheter is lubricated with petroleum jelly and gently inserted into the urethra until urine flow indicates its correct positioning within the bladder. A urine sample should be collected and sent for bacterial analysis. The bladder is drained until urine flow ceases and any residual volume should be documented. The catheter is then carefully taped into position and the external end connected to a giving set through which up to 500 ml of low iodine concentration water-soluble contrast agent is administered. The contrast agent is instilled under gravitational force using a slow drip-infusion technique, at approximately 8 ml/min[11] and continues until the child feels uncomfortably full or, in young children, spontaneous micturition occurs. Pulsed fluoroscopy is used periodically during contrast agent administration to check catheter position, bladder filling and the presence of ureteroceles or vesicoureteric reflux.

Spot images, as indicated in Table 5.5, may be taken with the patient supine or, alternatively, older children may be positioned erect.

**Table 5.5** Micturating cystourethrography projections.

| Timing and projection | Purpose |
| --- | --- |
| During early filling – PA[a] bladder | To check for ureteroceles |
| When bladder full – PA bladder | To assess bladder outline |
| During micturition: <br> Females:  PA urethra <br> Males:     45° oblique urethra | To check for urethral abnormalities (e.g. strictures). An oblique projection of the male urethra prevents radiographic foreshortening |
| During bladder filling and micturition – PA renal area | To check for vesicoureteric reflux |

[a] Postero-anterior.

# Summary

The role of radiography in the diagnosis of abdominal pathology is changing as alternative imaging modalities, particularly ultrasound, are increasingly used. However, plain film radiography and radiographic contrast agent examinations still have a role to play. This chapter has identified a number of clinical conditions where radiographic examinations may be beneficial in patient diagnosis and has provided advice to assist radiographers.

Guidance has also been offered on exposure factor selection and, if applied, this should maximise the chance of obtaining good quality radiographs and ensuring the radiation dose to the patient is keep as low as reasonably achievable.

# References

1. Sinclair, D. and Dangerfield, P. (1998) *Human Growth After Birth*, 6th edn. Oxford University Press, Oxford.
2. Marieb, E.N. (1992) *Human Anatomy and Physiology*, 2nd edn. The Benjamin/Cummings Publishing Company Inc, Redwood City.
3. Tortora, G.J. and Grabowski, S.A. (2000) *Principles of Anatomy and Physiology*, 9th edn. John Wiley & Sons Inc., New York.
4. Barr Lori, L. (ed.) (1991) *Handbook of Paediatric Imaging*. Churchill Livingstone, London.
5. Erkonen, W.E. (ed.) (1998) *Radiology 101: The Basics and Fundamentals of Imaging*. Lippincott-Raven, Philadelphia.
6. Behrman, R.E. and Kliegman, R.M. (eds) (1994) *Essentials of Pediatrics*, 2nd edn. W.B. Saunders Company, London.
7. Hull, D. and Johnston, D.I. (eds) (1999) *Essential Paediatrics*, 4th edn. Churchill Livingstone, London.
8. Buonomo, C. (2001) *Emergency Abdominal Conditions in Children*. Conference Proceedings of the Radiological Society of North America, 87th Scientific Assembly and Annual Meeting, November 25–30, 2001, Chicago, USA. Supplement to *Radiology* **221**, November 2001.
9. Royal College of Radiologists (1998) *Making the Best Use of a Department of Clinical Radiology: Guidelines for Doctors*, 4th edn. Royal College of Radiologists, London.
10. Cook, J.V., Pettet, A., Shah, K. *et al.* (1998) *Guidelines on Best Practice in the X-ray Imaging of Children: A Manual For All X-ray Departments*. Queen Mary's Hospital for Children, The St Helier NHS Trust, Carshalton, Surrey and The Radiological Protection Centre, St George's Healthcare NHS Trust, London.
11. Grainger, R.G., Allison, D.J., Adam, A. and Dixon, A.K. (2001) *Grainger and Allison's Diagnostic Radiology – A Textbook of Medical Imaging*, 4th edn. Churchill Livingstone, London.
12 Haller, J.O. and Slovis, T.L. (1995) *Pediatric Radiology*, 2nd edn. Springer, London.
13. Silverman, F.N. and Kuan, J.P. (1993) *Caffey's Pediatric X-Ray Diagnosis: An Integrated Imaging Approach*, 9th edn. Mosby, London.
14. Rennie, J.M. and Roberton, N.R.C. (1999) *Textbook of Neonatology*, 3rd edn. Churchill Livingstone, Edinburgh.

15. Gyll, C. and Blake, N. (1986) *Paediatric Diagnostic Imaging.* William Heinemann Medical Books, London.

16. Blickman, J.G. (1994) *Pediatric Radiology: The Requisites.* Mosby, London.

17. Kohn, M.M., Moores, B.M., Schibilla, H. *et al.* (eds) (1996) *European Guidelines on Quality Criteria for Diagnostic Radiographic Images in Paediatrics* (EUR 16261 EN). Office for Official Publications of the European Communities, Luxembourg.

18. Thompson, T.T. (1985) A *Practical Approach to Modern Imaging Equipment*, 2nd edn. Little, Brown and Company, Boston.

19. Carty, H., Shaw, D., Brunelle, F. and Kendall, B. (eds) (1994) *Imaging Children*, Volume 2. Churchill Livingstone, London.

20. Chapman, S. and Nakielny, R. (1993) *A Guide to Radiological Procedures*, 3rd edn. Baillière Tindall, London.

# Chapter 6
# Neonates

In order to produce high-quality radiographs of the neonate, the radiographer needs to be aware of special considerations relating to the care and safety of these patients. The aim of this chapter is to discuss technical factors and modifications to radiographic technique required for specific common neonatal pathologies and to highlight the particular demands of performing radiography in the neonatal care environment.

The neonatal period is classed as from the time of birth up to 28 days of age (Box 6.1). These first few days of independent life are a dangerous time for while neonatal mortality has consistently fallen, it still stands at around 4 per 1000 live births in the UK[2]. Neonatal deaths account for approximately 40% of all deaths in childhood[3] and it is therefore essential that newborn babies receive a high standard of care. Identifying those babies most at risk from neonatal morbidity and mortality is not an exact science, but gestational age at the time of birth and birthweight have been shown to be good indicators with the prognosis for very premature and extremely low birthweight babies being relatively poor despite significant improvements in survival rates over the last 20 years.

## Organisation of neonatal care

In the UK, the British Association of Perinatal Medicine recommends three categories of neonatal care as well as the accepted level of 'normal care'. These categories are:

(1) Special care
(2) High dependency or level 2 intensive care
(3) Intensive care or level 1 intensive care

The level of medical intervention and care received by the neonate increases within these clinical categories with level 1 intensive care being appropriate for those neonates who are most at risk or require frequent medical intervention. Level 1 intensive care is therefore often provided within regional paediatric centres where specialist knowledge, experience and expertise in neonatal genetics, surgery and radiology are greater. In contrast, special care, and in many instances level 2 intensive care, are generally provided within district hospitals.

**Box 6.1**   Terms associated with neonates.

Early neonatal period:   birth to 7 days
Late neonatal period:   7 days to 28 days
Post neonatal period:   from 28 days to 1 year of age
Perinatal period:   the period shortly before or after birth
Infant:   first year of life
Term:   from 37 to less than 42 completed weeks gestation
Pre-term:   less than 37 completed weeks of gestation[1]
Post-term:   42 weeks or more gestation
Low birthweight:   less than 2500 g at full gestation
Very low birthweight:   birthweight less than 1500 g
Extremely low birthweight:   birthweight less than 1000 g

# Care by the radiographer

Neonatal radiography requires the radiographer to have not only a high level of technical expertise, but also an understanding of important aspects of neonatal care and the following points, related to handling, infection, warmth and noise, are intended to raise the radiographer's awareness of non-radiographic aspects of neonatal patient care.

## *Handling*

Touching and holding a new baby is important for the psychological welfare of the guardians and the child. However, episodes of bradycardia, hypoxia, apnoea and disturbance of sleep patterns are all associated with handling. These factors, combined with the increased risk of heat loss, cross-infection and the possibility of damage to the delicate skin of a pre-term baby, mean that handling by the radiographer should be kept to a minimum and the assistance of the nursing staff or guardians sought.

## *Infection*

All newborn babies, particularly those born prematurely, are susceptible to infection as a result of their defensive mechanisms being underdeveloped (Box 6.2). This immunodeficiency increases the risk of systemic spread of contracted infections which, if left untreated, may lead to septicaemic shock and neonatal mortality[4]. Any neonate suspected of having an infection should therefore be treated with antibiotics.

The radiographer can reduce the risk of neonatal infection by undertaking the following measures:

- Removing wrist watches and jewellery that may come into contact with the neonate prior to hand washing.

**Box 6.2**   Infection defence mechanisms.

> *Physical defences*:   The skin acts as a natural physical barrier to infection but its defences are reduced during the neonatal period as the skin is delicate, easily damaged and lacks the normal non-pathogenic bacteria that in themselves provide protection. Necrosis of the umbilical stump can also act as a focus for infection as can medical intervention and the introduction of catheters, endotracheal and naso-gastric tubes.
>
> *Humoral immunity*:   Humoral immunity relates to the production of antibodies by the body to combat bacteria or viruses. Certain of these antibodies may be deficient in the neonate.
>
> *Phagocyte function*:   The phagocytic function of leucocytes is reduced during the neonatal period.

- Hand washing with an antibacterial agent prior to, and following, the radiographic examination; elbow taps and paper towels should be used in preference to hand taps and warm air dryers to minimise the risk of cross-infection but the wearing of gowns, gloves or masks is not routinely advocated as there is no evidence that their use decreases the risk of cross-infection[1].
- Cleaning cassettes and other accessory equipment that may come into contact with the neonate prior to examination.
- Covering the equipment with clean linen (e.g. a pillowcase) will also reduce neonatal heat loss.

Where possible, radiographers who are suffering from viral infections (e.g. herpes simplex) should not undertake neonatal radiography. If this is unavoidable, then increased attention should be given to measures designed to minimise cross-infection, in particular hand-washing[2].

## Warmth

The pre-term neonate has difficulty in maintaining adequate body temperature as a result of having a relatively large surface area compared to body weight, and an inability to produce heat by shivering. As a consequence, the neonate is susceptible to heat loss and its associated clinical complications (e.g. reduced surfactant synthesis and efficiency, postnatal weight loss, increased oxygen consumption, hypoglycaemia and increased mortality). To address this issue, neonates are generally nursed fully clothed unless this is prohibited by medical treatment (e.g. phototherapy), and radiographers should ensure that only essential handling and undressing of the neonate occurs in order to maintain neonatal body temperature. Additional precautions of warming or covering all objects that may come into direct contact with the neonate (e.g. cassettes) and performing the radiographic examination, where possible, within the neonate's own environment (e.g. within the incubator) should also be taken.

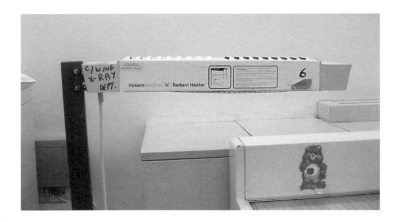

**Fig. 6.1**  A radiant warmer.

Neonatal in-patients who are particularly at risk from heat loss may be nursed beneath a radiant warmer and this may need to be removed during radiographic examination to facilitate the positioning of the x-ray tube. Radiographers should ensure that the length of time the heater is removed is minimised and that the heater is replaced upon completion of the examination. Neonates examined within the radiology department are still susceptible to heat loss and a convector heater should be available within the imaging department to enable the examination room to be warmed. Alternatively, departments undertaking a large volume of neonatal examinations may employ a radiant warmer (Fig. 6.1).

### Noise

Sudden loud noises can precipitate sleep disturbance, crying, tachycardia, hypoxaemia and raised intracranial pressure[1] in the neonate and as a result it is recommended that noise levels within the incubator should not exceed 45 decibels[5]. Possible sources of loud noise for a neonate nursed within an incubator are objects being placed on the incubator roof and closure of the incubator doors.

## Respiratory and cardiovascular pathology

Respiratory difficulty or distress frequently presents during the neonatal period and has a variety of causes. An important factor in the differential diagnosis of underlying pathology is the time at which symptoms of respiratory distress occur[2] (Table 6.1).

### Transient tachypnoea

Transient tachypnoea of the newborn is an ill-defined but common condition thought to result from a delay in the clearing of amniotic fluid from the lungs[6]. Symptoms typically manifest within 3 hours of birth and a clinical diagnosis is

**Table 6.1**   Common causes of neonatal respiratory difficulty.

| Onset: birth–6 hours | Onset: >6 hours post-delivery | Onset: any time after birth |
|---|---|---|
| • Transient tachypnoea<br>• Hyaline membrane disease<br>• Meconium aspiration<br>• Pneumothorax<br>• Persistent pulmonary hypertension<br>• Congenital malformations | • Pneumonia<br>• Congenital heart disease<br>• Underlying metabolic illness | • Upper airway obstruction<br>• Neurological disorders |

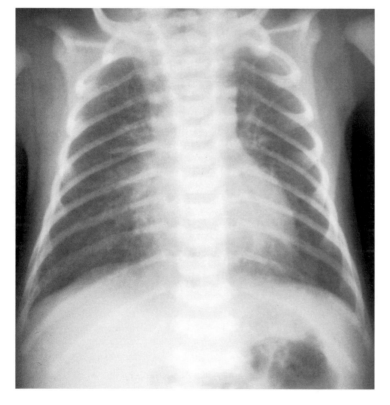

**Fig. 6.2**   Transient tachypnoea.

possible where the respiratory rate exceeds 60/min[1]. Chest radiography undertaken within a few hours of birth may show evidence of hyperinflation, pleural effusion, fluid within the fissures, streaky opacification and prominent vascular markings[6] (Fig. 6.2). However, these radiographic findings are also consistent with neonatal pneumonia and further radiographic examinations may be required to monitor the progress of the condition. Complete clinical and radiographic resolution of transient tachypnoea should occur within 24 hours.

## Hyaline membrane disease (idiopathic respiratory distress syndrome – IRDS)

Hyaline membrane disease (HMD) is an acute respiratory illness that results from a lack of surfactant within the neonatal lungs. Surfactant diminishes alveolar surface tension thereby preventing atelectasis (collapse) of the alveoli and acini and assisting in the maintenance of normal respiratory function. The incidence of HMD is directly related to gestational age at the time of birth[7] with very pre-term babies being most at risk. Clinical symptoms of HMD include cyanosis, tachypnoea, expiratory 'grunting' and intercostal retraction[8]. Regular radiographic assessment is likely to be requested to monitor the progress of the disease. Radiographically, the lungs are under-inflated and appear opaque or mottled, although air bronchograms may be evident (Fig. 6.3). Treatment is dependent upon the underlying causative condition.

## Meconium aspiration

Meconium is a dark green discharge that results from the 'sloughing off' of dead bowel wall cells during foetal development. It is contained within the intestines of the full-term foetus and is usually passed within 24 hours of delivery. However, if foetal distress should occur during delivery then evacuation of meconium into the amniotic fluid may occur and in a small amount of cases (1%), aspiration of the meconium will result[8] causing respiratory obstruction (air trapping) and distress. Radiographic examination of the neonatal chest will reveal hyperinflated lungs and patchy, bilateral opacification[2] which may become more diffuse as the condition progresses (Fig. 6.4). Clinically, symptoms of respiratory distress as a result of meconium aspiration resolve within 3–5 days of delivery although radiographic resolution may take up to 1 year.

## Pulmonary interstitial emphysema

Surfactant deficiency in the premature neonate may result in the rupture of small airways and dissection of air into the interstitial space where it forms small cysts within the interlobular septae (pulmonary interstitial emphysema). The neonate may present asymptomatically or display signs of gradual degeneration and progressive hypoxaemia if the condition is diffuse. Radiographic evidence of the condition includes areas of translucency and atelectasis (collapse).

## Pneumothorax

Pneumothorax is a common complication of ventilator therapy, particularly if high pressures have been used. If the pneumothorax is large then the neonate will suffer respiratory difficulty and display signs of general deterioration. In these circumstances, a clinical diagnosis can be made following physical examination. In contrast, small pneumothoraces may be asymptomatic and remain undetected until discovered incidentally on a chest radiograph. Radiological

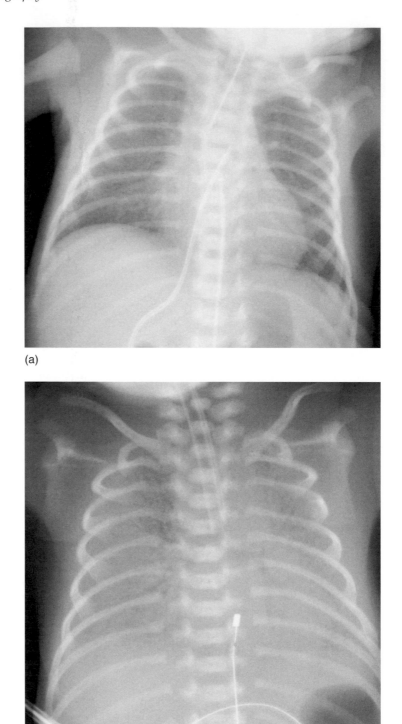

(a)

(b)

**Fig. 6.3**   (a) and (b) Hyaline membrane disease.

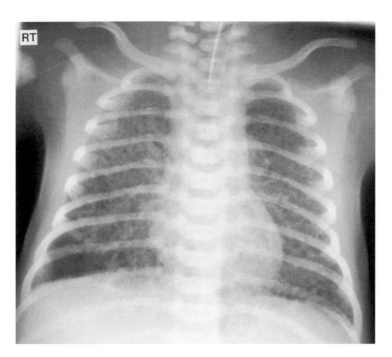

**Fig. 6.4** Meconium aspiration.

signs of a pneumothorax are the absence of lung markings peripherally within the thoracic cavity and increased opacification of the affected lung (Figs 6.5–6.8). In cases where radiological diagnosis is uncertain, a horizontal beam lateral chest projection with the patient supine may be undertaken to demonstrate retrosternal air (Fig. 6.6). However, the radiographer must remember to reduce the selected kV and mAs appropriately to prevent over exposure of the retrosternal region.

## Pneumomediastinum

Pneumomediastinum (air within the mediastinal cavity) is commonly asymptomatic and has a variety of causative agents (e.g. severe asthma or excessive resuscitation). It can be recognised on the antero-posterior chest radiograph as a 'halo' of air adjacent to the heart borders (Fig. 6.9) and, in cases of uncertainty, a horizontal beam lateral chest radiograph is useful to demonstrate marked retrosternal hyperlucency[3].

## Pneumopericardium

Pneumopericardium in the pre-term infant may occur as a complication of mechanical ventilation and can be identified radiographically as a hyperlucent cardiac shadow (Fig. 6.10). Clinically, the child may display signs of pallor, shock and hypotension as a result of cardiac tamponade[3].

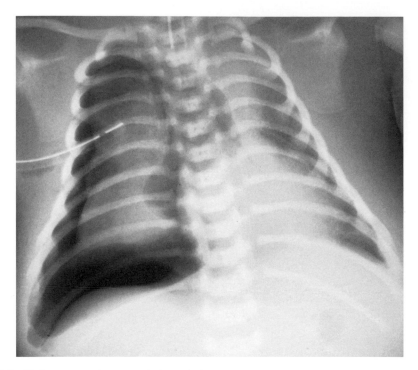

**Fig. 6.5**   Right pneumothorax and chest drain.

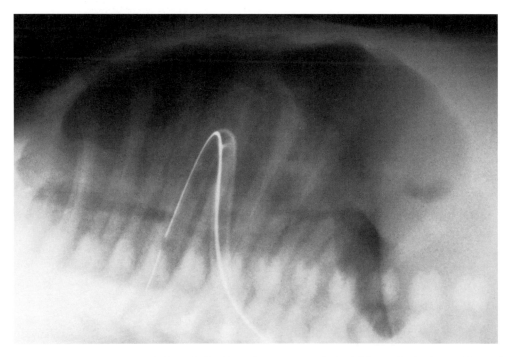

**Fig. 6.6**   Right pneumothorax and chest drain. Note the retrosternal air visible on the horizontal beam lateral projection.

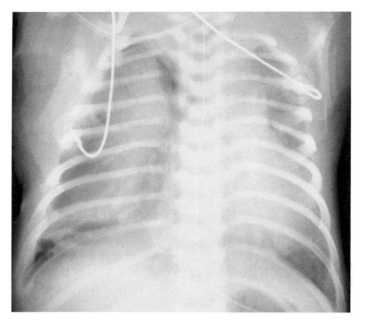

**Fig. 6.7** Pneumothorax with hyaline membrane disease.

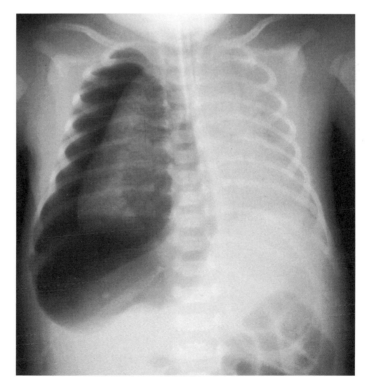

**Fig. 6.8** Tension pneumothorax.

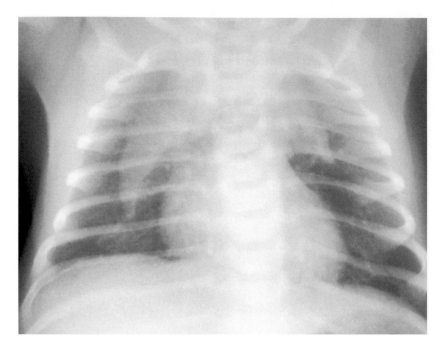

**Fig. 6.9**   Pneumomediastinum.

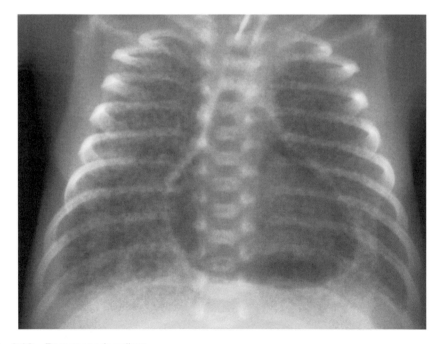

**Fig. 6.10**   Pneumopericardium.

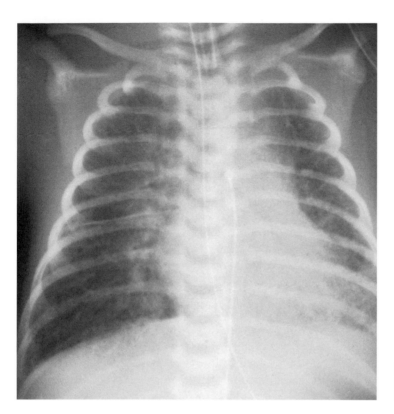

**Fig. 6.11** Neonatal pneumonia. Patchy consolidation throughout both lung fields.

## Pneumonia

Pneumonia is the inflammation of the lungs due to infection and, in neonates, the causative agent is generally bacterial rather than viral. The infection is often acquired at the time of delivery, possibly from the amniotic fluid or birth canal, but it may also occur as a consequence of intubation and ventilation. The clinical and radiographic signs of neonatal pneumonia are non-specific and the antero-posterior chest radiograph will demonstrate ill-defined perihilar and pulmonary opacification[3] (Fig. 6.11). Failure to treat neonatal pneumonia may result in neonatal fatality and therefore all neonates displaying signs of respiratory distress without a clear non-infective cause should be treated routinely with antibiotics.

## Congenital malformations

Congenital abnormalities associated with the respiratory system are rare but can give rise to respiratory difficulties. Examples of congenital abnormalities include: diaphragmatic hernia (see Chapter 5); congenital lobar emphysema, where radiography may demonstrate the overaeration of a single pulmonary lobe[9]; pulmonary hypoplasia, which results in overdevelopment of the unaffected lung/lobes; and choanal atresia, a structural abnormality of the posterior nasopharynx. Plain film radiography of the chest and upper respiratory tract may be helpful in the diagnosis of all these conditions.

## Persistent pulmonary hypertension

Persistent pulmonary hypertension (PPHN) occurs when foetal circulation persists after birth. Clinical symptoms include cyanosis and occasionally respiratory distress, for which diagnostic chest radiography may be requested. Persistent pulmonary hypertension is associated with a variety of structural cardiac abnormalities[3] and the radiographic appearances of the condition are therefore dependent upon the underlying cause.

## Congenital heart disease

Congenital heart disease presents in approximately 1 in 100 live births[4] and may be structural or functional in nature. The accurate diagnosis of neonatal cardiac disease is essential if early medical and surgical intervention is to be undertaken. However, plain film radiography is not specific in the diagnosis of congenital heart disease and therefore radiographic results need to be correlated with clinical findings, laboratory tests and other cardiac imaging[10] (Fig. 6.12), in particular echocardiography[9]. Clinical symptoms of congenital heart disease are also dependent upon the nature of the condition, and therefore classification of congenital heart disease is often based upon the presence or absence of cyanosis[10] (Tables 6.2 and 6.3).

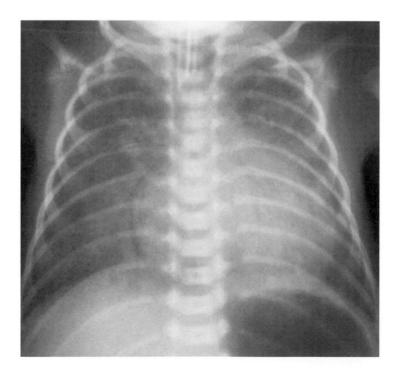

**Fig. 6.12**  Several cardiac abnormalities co-existing. Note enlarged heart.

**Table 6.2**   Radiographic appearance of cyanotic congenital heart disease.

| Cyanotic defect | Radiographic appearances |
|---|---|
| Tetralogy of Fallot | Heart size normal; elevated cardiac apex; right-sided aortic arch (25% cases) |
| Pulmonary stenosis | Heart enlarged; elevated cardiac apex |
| Transposition of the Great Vessels | Heart size initially normal – enlarges over time; thymus small or absent |
| Tricuspid atresia | Heart size normal; associated with other malformations; radiographic appearances varied |
| Persistent truncus arteriosus | Pronounced truncus; heart enlarged; elevated cardiac apex; right-sided aorta (25% cases) |
| Total anomalous pulmonary venous return (TAPVR) | Cardiac enlargement (right-sided) |

**Table 6.3**   Radiographic appearance of acyanotic congenital heart disease.

| Acyanotic defect | Radiographic appearances |
|---|---|
| Patent ductus arteriosus | Slight cardiac enlargement; commonest cardiac cause of respiratory distress[9] |
| Interatrial septal defect | Slight cardiac enlargement possible (right atrium and ventricle) |
| Ventricular septal defect | Most common congenital condition; heart enlarged; aorta normal size |
| Coarctation of aorta | Narrowing of aorta at site of coarctation; rib notching seen in older children but not in those under 5 years of age[10] |

### Pierre Robin syndrome

Pierre Robin syndrome consists of three co-existing abnormalities: small lower jaw, midline cleft palate and the abnormal attachment of the genioglossi muscles. As a result of these abnormalities, the tongue is displaced backwards, obstructing the oropharynx and producing respiratory problems. Pneumonia is a common complication of this syndrome and plain film radiography of the chest may be requested to assist in the diagnosis. However, in order to reduce the risk of respiratory obstruction by the tongue, these patients are usually nursed prone and the radiographic examination should be undertaken in the presenting position where possible.

## Abdominal pathology

Indications for neonatal abdominal radiography typically relate to pathologies of the gastrointestinal or renal tract and many of these conditions will have been recognised sonographically during the antenatal period. As a result, many neonatal imaging examinations are required to assess the extent of a condition or assist in treatment planning rather than provide a primary diagnosis.

## Bowel atresia

Bowel atresia is the commonest cause of bowel obstruction in neonates. The radiographic appearances of atresia vary according to the level at which the atresia occurs (Box 6.3) but a common feature of all presentations is the absence of bowel gas distal to the site of the atresia and a dilated bowel proximal to it.

**Box 6.3**    Bowel atresia.

*Oesophageal atresia* (Figs 6.13–6.15)
- Affects 1 in 3500 live births
- Failure of the oesophagus to connect to rest of gastrointestinal tract
- Classified into five types – many involve a tracheal fistula
- 50% of neonates with this condition have co-existing abnormalities[11]
- Aspiration pneumonia a frequent complication
- An antero-posterior radiograph of the chest and upper abdomen following insertion of a radio-opaque tube may be required to identify site of atresia. In a complete atresia the tip of the tube will be seen to lie in the oesophagus and no gas will be seen in the abdomen. If gas is visible within the abdomen then this suggests a tracheo-oesophageal fistula

*Duodenal atresia* (Fig. 6.16)
- Failure of the duodenum to connect to the distal gastrointestinal tract
- Affects 1 in 6000 live births
- 30% of cases are associated with Down's syndrome[2]
- An abdominal radiograph will demonstrate a large amount of gas in the stomach and duodenum but no gas in the distal gastrointestinal tract ('double bubble' sign)

*Jejunal and ileal atresia*
- Commonly a congenital stenosis rather than a complete atresia that generally causes obstruction in later infancy rather than during the neonatal period
- No known associated pathologies or conditions
- Radiographic appearances are typical of small bowel obstruction with dilated loops of small bowel and fluid levels being visible

Anorectal atresia (imperforate anus)
- Congenital lack of continuity between rectum and anus
- An inverted erect lateral projection of the pelvis may occasionally be taken using a horizontal x-ray beam

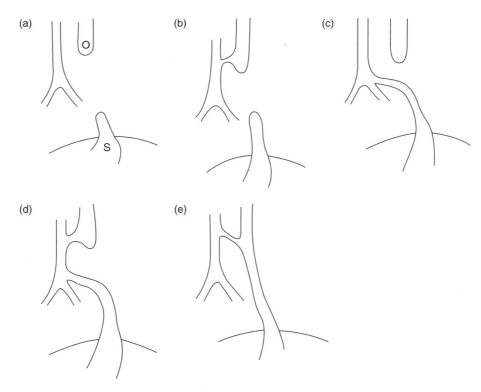

**Fig. 6.13** Diagram depicting the five variations of oesophageal atresia. (a) Atresia – no fistula (5–10%). (b) Oesophageal atresia with high fistula only (1%). (c) Oesophageal atresia with low fistula only (80–90%). (d) Oesophageal fistula with low and high fistula (2–3%). (e) H-fistula with no atresia (5–8%). o = oesophagus; s = stomach.

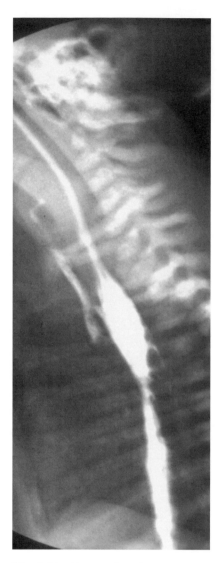

**Fig. 6.14** H-type of tracheo-oesophageal atresia.

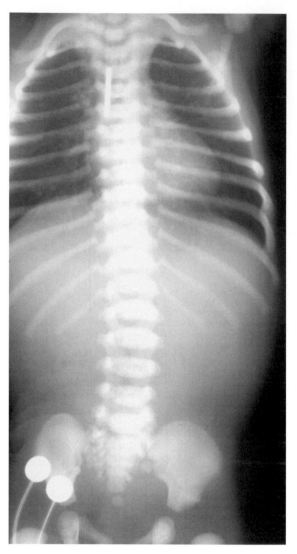

**Fig. 6.15** Oesophageal atresia. Total absence of gas in the bowel.

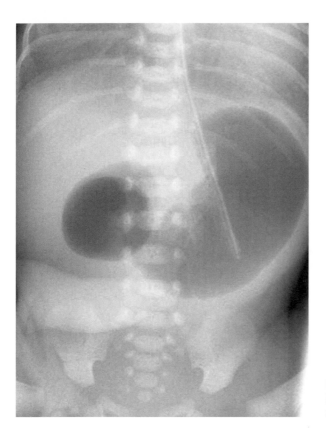

**Fig. 6.16** Duodenal atresia. Note the 'double bubble' sign and the absence of gas in distal gastrointestinal tract.

## Malrotation

Malrotation occurs when the bowel fails to take up its normal position during embryonic development. Clinical symptoms of malrotation are often intermittent in nature and vary with the severity of the condition (e.g. the patient may be asymptomatic or may present with severe duodenal obstruction or volvulus). Plain film abdominal radiographs are generally unremarkable, although some may show an abnormal distribution of bowel gas (Fig. 6.17). A contrast meal is the diagnostic examination of choice (Fig. 6.18).

## Volvulus

A volvulus is a twisting of the bowel around its long axis leading to obstruction. Failure to accurately diagnose and treat a volvulus can lead to bowel infarction[12] and necrosis as a consequence of compression of the mesenteric vessels. As a result, a volvulus is a surgical emergency. Radiographic demonstration of a volvulus is dependent upon the severity of the condition and, although plain film abdominal radiographs may demonstrate abnormally positioned bowel or duodenal obstruction, an upper gastrointestinal contrast study is the examination of choice for diagnosis[9].

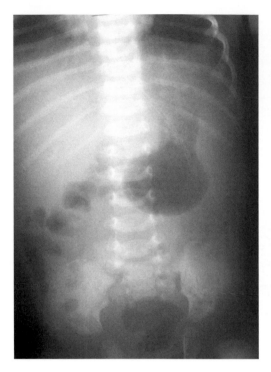

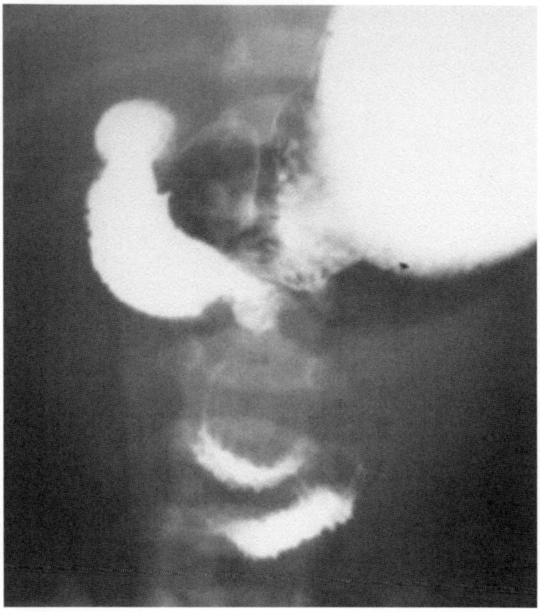

**Fig. 6.18**   Contrast examination demonstrating malrotation.

**Fig. 6.17**   Plain film of the abdomen on a patient with malrotation.

## Meconium ileus

A meconium ileus is a form of distal intestinal obstruction caused by dry, thickened meconium at the terminal ileum. Abdominal radiography will demonstrate marked bowel distension proximal to the obstruction and possibly a coarse, granular bowel mass at the site of the meconium ileus (Fig. 6.19). It is thought that the majority of patients presenting with this condition will have cystic fibrosis (>90% of cases)[9]. Where diagnostic uncertainty exists, ultrasound may accurately differentiate between meconium ileus and ileal atresia. In all other cases, the use of a water-soluble, iodine-based ionic contrast agent enema is the diagnostic, and possibly therapeutic, examination of choice. However, this type of enema has an associated risk of bowel perforation and therefore should only be performed within specialist paediatric centres[9].

## Meconium plug

A meconium plug is a form of large bowel obstruction that results from the failure of meconium to pass through the large bowel as a consequence of colonic inertia. A plain abdominal radiograph may demonstrate the obstruction as multiple air-filled, distended loops of bowel. A warmed enema of a water-soluble, iodined-based ionic contrast agent is the examination of choice to assist in diagnosis and promote the passage of the meconium.

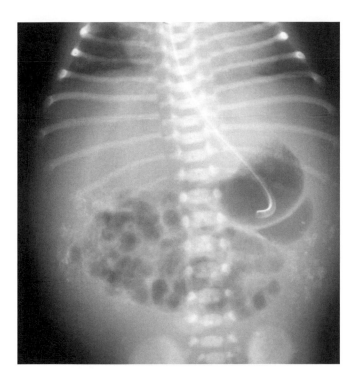

**Fig. 6.19** Meconium ileus.

## *Congenital megacolon (Hirschprung's disease)*

The congenital absence of ganglionic nerve cells in the wall of the colon results in a complete or partial functional obstruction and dilation of the large bowel as a consequence of peristaltic failure. Congenital megacolon accounts for 10–20% of all neonatal intestinal obstructions and may be associated with perforation (5% of cases). The plain abdominal radiograph may demonstrate a distal colonic obstruction with extremely dilated bowel proximal to it.

## *Necrotising enterocolitis*

Necrotising enterocolitis (NEC) is a progressive inflammatory disease of the bowel commonly associated with prematurity (85% of cases developing in neonates of less than 37 weeks gestational age[13]). The exact aetiology of the condition is unknown. However, infection, maternal substance abuse and umbilical cannulation are all associated with an increased risk of NEC[9]. Clinical symptoms are initially non-specific but as the disease progresses abdominal distension, bilious vomiting, bloody stools, intestinal obstruction and perforation of the bowel wall may be noted. Abdominal radiographs in the initial stages of the disease are non-specific demonstrating minimal gastric or bowel distension. As the condition progresses, greater distension of the bowel, air in the bowel wall (pneumatosis intestinalis) and pneumoperitoneum as a result of bowel perforation (30% of cases) may be seen (Figs 6.20 and 6.21). Plain film radiography of the abdomen may be requested in order to monitor the progress of the

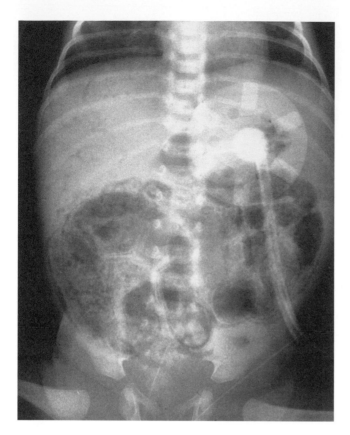

**Fig. 6.20**  Necrotising enterocolitis. Bowel distension, pneumatosis intestinalsis and pneumoperitoneum.

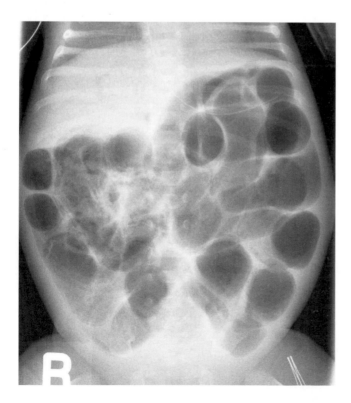

**Fig. 6.21**  Necrotising enterocolitis. Note the significant bowel distension.

condition. However, ultrasound may also have a role to play in the assessment of suspected pneumatosis intestinalis. Contrast studies are not indicated during the acute phase but a contrast enema may be undertaken at follow-up to demonstrate any resultant bowel strictures[13].

### Abdominal mass

An abdominal mass is identified in approximately 1 in every 1000 live births[14] and, during the neonatal period, these are most frequently associated with renal tract abnormalities (see Chapter 5). In all circumstances, ultrasound is the imaging modality of choice for primary investigations.

### Jaundice

Neonatal jaundice may result from a variety of physiological and metabolic causes, most of which can be successfully treated medically without the need for imaging. Prolonged neonatal jaundice (>7–10 days) is a common indication for urgent ultrasound imaging of the neonatal liver, primarily to exclude biliary atresia[9] (partial or complete congenital interruption of the common bile duct[12]).

## Catheters, lines and tubes

Many neonatal radiographic examinations are undertaken to assess the position of lines and catheters prior to their medical use and it is important that radiographers are able to identify incorrectly positioned catheters and bring these findings to the attention of their radiological and medical colleagues.

### Endotracheal tube

Endotracheal intubation is necessary for mechanical ventilation, and accurate positioning of the endotracheal tube within the trachea is essential if effective ventilation is to be achieved and respiratory obstruction avoided. The distal tip of the tube should be positioned at the level of the second thoracic vertebra, approximately 1 – 2 cm above the carina[2]. It is important, when undertaking plain film radiography to assess the position of the endotracheal tube, that the baby's head is in its natural position (i.e. that position in which it is being nursed), as movement of the head can alter the position of the endotracheal tube and the radiographic location of the distal tip will therefore not be consistent with the actual location of the tube (Fig. 6.22).

### Umbilical arterial catheter

Catheterisation of the umbilical artery provides a secure access for the invasive monitoring of blood and the infusion of fluids. On entry at the umbilicus the arterial catheter should initially run caudally towards the pelvis before entering

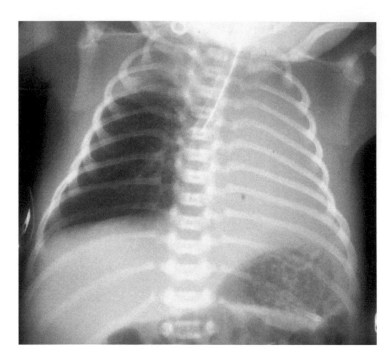

**Fig. 6.22**  Incorrectly positioned endotracheal tube. Note the tip is at the level of T5 resulting in collapse of the left lung.

the internal iliac artery and ascending the aorta (Fig. 6.23). A correctly positioned umbilical arterial catheter should lie in the lower aorta (below vertebra L3) or above the diaphragm (higher than vertebra T12) in order to avoid the renal arteries as they exit from the aorta. Plain film radiography to assess the position of the arterial catheter should include both the chest and abdomen in order to demonstrate its entire length.

### Umbilical venous catheter

When correctly positioned, the umbilical venous catheter should be seen running cranially from the umbilicus along the umbilical vein, the ductus venosus and the inferior vena cava to lie with its tip within the right atrium of the heart (Fig. 6.23). It is used primarily to deliver drugs and fluids and to monitor central venous pressures. Plain film radiography to assess the position of the catheter should include the chest and upper abdomen (from the level of the umbilicus) to ensure that the entire length of the catheter is visualised.

### Central venous catheter

Central venous catheters are inserted into the veins of the antecubital fossa, the long saphenous vein or the superficial temporal

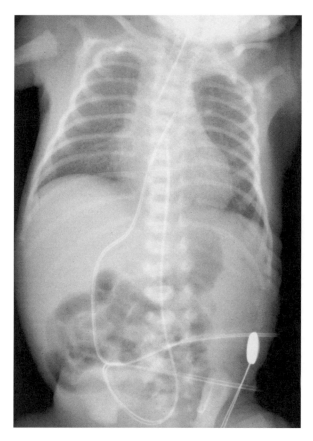

**Fig. 6.23** Umbilical arterial and venous catheters *in situ*. Note how the arterial catheter runs caudally initially before turning to run cranially with the aorta.

veins. When correctly positioned the tip should lie at the junction of the superior vena cava and the right atrium.

## Chest drain

A chest drain is normally sited following identification of a pneumothorax (Fig. 6.5). Common insertion sites are the anterior chest wall through the second or third intercostal spaces directly lateral to the mid-clavicular line, and the lateral chest wall through the fourth, fifth or sixth intercostal spaces directly anterior to the axillary line. The tube should be inserted approximately 3 cm into the thoracic cavity and directed towards the apex of the lung. A chest drain may also be used to drain collections of plural fluid, in which case the tube usually requires directing posteriorly and inferiorly[15].

### Feeding tubes

Orogastric or nasogastric feeding tubes are used as an alternative to intravenous feeding when normal gastric feeding is inappropriate. In addition, they may also facilitate gastric or small bowel decompression in cases of excessive abdominal distension. When correctly positioned, the tip of the nasogastric/orogastric tube should be identified within the stomach or, where a nasojejunal feeding tube is used, within the jejunum.

## Radiographic technique for the chest

### Antero-posterior (supine)

The antero-posterior supine chest radiograph is the most common neonatal chest projection. However, its production is fraught with difficulties.

A clean sheet or a pillowcase should be used to cover the cassette in order to reduce the risk of cross-infection and prevent neonatal heat loss when in contact with a cold surface. Check if an apnoea mattress is being used. If it is then care should be taken not to place the cassette under the mattress, as it may be visible on the resultant radiograph. If the neonate is placed directly onto a covered cassette then the apnoea alarm will need to be deactivated and then reset when the cassette is removed.

The neonate's arms should be flexed on either side of the head and the head held straight to prevent rotation. Care must be taken to avoid extending the arms as this may result in lordosis. If the neonate is quiet it may be possible to prop the head straight and to leave the arms abducted. This will avoid any irradiation to the health care worker who would otherwise be required to immobilise the patient. To avoid a lordotic projection a 15° pad should be used or, alternatively, the incubator tray could be angled with the head end raised 15°. Care must also be taken to ensure the chin does not obscure the upper chest; this can be achieved by placing a small pillow or roll of cotton wool under the neck. If the neonate is intubated then the head will probably be turned to the side. In this case the head should not be straightened but left in the presenting position as straightening the head may cause the distal end of the endotracheal tube to move slightly which may be significant if the radiograph is required to assess tube position. It is important that the pelvis is also straight to reduce rotation. A rolled blanket placed under the legs may help to immobilise the neonate in the correct position.

The neonate should be positioned in the incubator so as to avoid any curves/cut-outs in the incubator roof that may be visible on the resultant radiograph and detract from the quality of the film (Fig. 6.24) and, where possible, wires and tubes should be moved from the area of interest.

Lead rubber should be placed on top of the incubator to provide protection to the neonate abdomen and head. Many intensive care units use small intensive care beds rather than incubators in order to facilitate easy access to the neonate

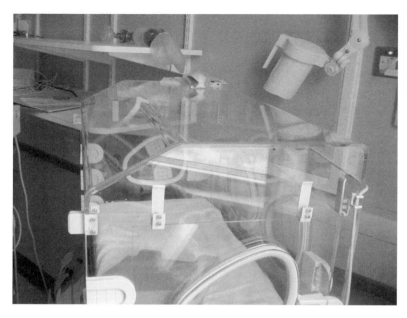

**Fig. 6.24** A typical incubator with a curved roof. The curve must be excluded from the projection or it will be visible on the radiograph.

for medical and nursing staff. In these instances protection for the head can be applied by use of a lead rubber glove and an additional lead shield held over the neonate (Fig. 6.25).

The x-ray beam should be perpendicular to the cassette and centred to the middle of the sternum with lower collimation at a level just above the lower costal margin.

The exposure should be made on normal inspiration. Neonates are abdominal breathers and therefore the rise and fall of the abdomen is a good indicator of the phase of respiration – inspiration being indicated when the abdomen is rising. It is essential to obtain an adequately inspired radiograph in order to optimise the visualisation of lung tissue and enable accurate assessment of the cardiac size and shape. If the neonate becomes distressed then the radiographer should wait to expose the film until the neonate has ceased crying. If the child is radiographed whilst crying then the lungs can appear overinflated and this hyperinflation can mimic pathology. An exposure time of less than 4 ms[16] should be used in order to avoid recorded movement unsharpness resulting from rapid heart and respiratory movement. In order to achieve this short exposure time and deliver the required mAs, a relatively high-powered mobile unit must be used. All exposure factors (Box 6.4), including the mobile used, should be recorded on the film together with the date and time of exposure.

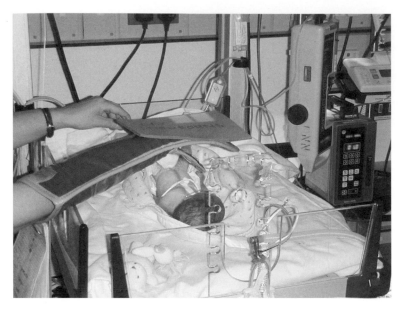

**Fig. 6.25**  Lead protection of neonate nursed in open top incubator.

**Box 6.4** Exposure factors – neonatal chest radiography. (Adapted from European Guidelines[16].)

| | |
|---|---|
| Nominal focal spot value: | 0.6 mm |
| Focus-to-film distance (FFD): | 80–100 cm |
| Kilovoltage: | 60–65 kV |
| Exposure time: | < 4 ms |
| Film-screen system: | nominal speed class 200–400 |
| Additional filtration: | up to 1 mm Al + 0.1 or 0.2 mm Cu (or equivalent) |
| Anti-scatter grid: | none |

If the neonate is being nursed prone then the radiograph should be taken in this position to minimise patient handling. However, be aware that the prone position results in rotation of the thorax and compensatory padding may need to be placed beneath the patient.

A single antero-posterior supine radiograph of the chest and abdomen together should only be performed on *small* neonates when checking the position of lines and tubes (e.g. umbilical arterial catheter). The positioning and centring should be as for a chest x-ray but the collimation should be adjusted to include the symphysis pubis. This positioning and centring is adopted to ensure that the resultant chest image is of diagnostic quality (i.e. not lordotic in appearance) but care must be taken to ensure that the head is adequately protected. It should also be noted that due to the divergent nature of the x-ray beam the position of lines and tubes on the radiograph may not be an accurate representation of their true position.

The neonatal chest radiograph should be of good technical quality as technical errors can mimic or mask significant pathologies. The criteria for judging the technical quality of a chest radiograph are discussed in Chapter 4.

## Lateral chest

A lateral projection may be needed to confirm a suspected radiological diagnosis (Box 6.5) and this can be taken in either the lateral decubitus or supine decubitus position (Fig. 6.26). The position of the incubator apertures should be considered when choosing the most appropriate projection in order to avoid artefacts on the image. In addition, the supine decubitus may have the advantage that it is less likely to involve changing the patient's position.

**Box 6.5**  Pathologies that may require a lateral chest radiograph.

- Pneumothorax (results in free air in pleural space)
- Plural effusion (results in free fluid in pleural space)
- Abnormality of the thoracic cage
- Abnormality of the diaphragm
- Congenital cardiac abnormality
- Chest mass
- Collapse

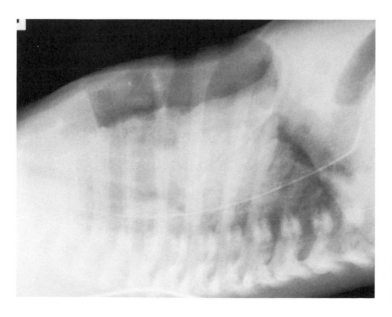

**Fig. 6.26**  Lateral chest radiograph with the patient in the supine decubitus position. There is evidence of a pneumothorax.

### *Antero-posterior in the lateral decubitus position*

If free air or fluid is suspected in the pleural space then an antero-posterior chest radiograph, with the neonate in the lateral decubitus position, may be necessary. The neonate should be positioned on radiolucent sponge pads with the affected side down if free fluid is suspected (in order to identify fluid levels) or affected side raised if free air is suspected (Fig. 6.27).

# Radiographic technique for the abdomen and related anatomy

### *Antero-posterior (supine)*

As in the adult, this projection is the routine projection taken for the abdomen. However, there are differences that the radiographer should be aware of. The anatomical shape of an infant's abdomen varies from that of the adult in that it is essentially as wide as it is long, with thin abdominal walls and therefore the abdominal organs can be eccentric in position (Fig. 6.28). As a result of this difference in abdominal shape, care needs to be taken with collimation to prevent over-collimation and exclusion of the lateral abdominal walls and the upper abdomen. A useful centring point is in the midline at a level just below the lower costal margin. Lead rubber protection should be used to protect the thighs, upper chest and head.

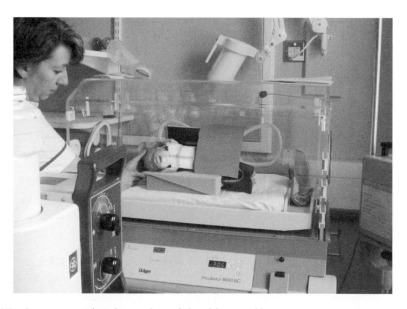

**Fig. 6.27**   Antero-posterior chest – lateral decubitus position.

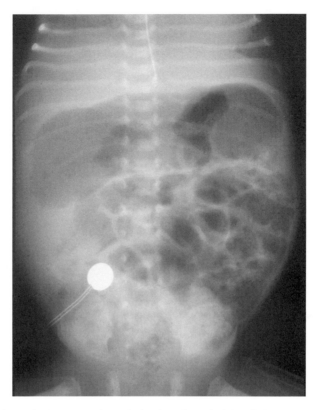

**Fig. 6.28** Radiograph demonstrating relative length and width of abdomen, the thin abdominal walls and small pelvis.

### Lateral abdomen (supine)

This projection is useful for demonstrating fluid levels within the gastrointestinal tract or detecting signs of perforation (i.e. free air within the abdominal cavity).

The lateral projection of the abdomen with the neonate in the supine position has been suggested to be the most useful projection for demonstrating free air in cases of perforation[17]. The perforation will result in small triangles of gas visible against the anterior abdominal wall (Fig. 6.29). If possible the neonate should be raised to lie on a covered radiolucent sponge in order to ensure that the posterior abdominal wall is included. The median sagittal plane should be parallel to a vertically supported cassette and the neonate positioned as close to the cassette as possible (Fig. 6.30). The resultant radiographs should include the whole of the abdomen from the diaphragm to the ischial tuberosities.

### Antero-posterior lateral decubitus abdomen

The antero-posterior projection, with the neonate in the lateral decubitus position, is also a useful projection for demonstrating fluid levels within the gastrointestinal tract or for detecting signs of perforation. In cases of perforation the neonate should be laid on their left side to prevent free air being masked by, or confused with, air within the stomach. The resultant radiograph should include the whole of the abdomen including the rectal region and lateral abdominal walls. To achieve this the neonate should be placed on a covered foam sponge

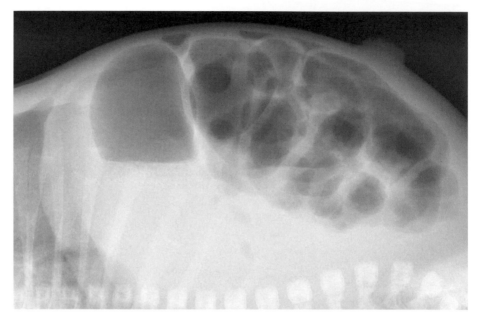

**Fig. 6.29** Lateral abdominal projection with the patient in the supine position. Note the free interperitoneal air (triangle sign).

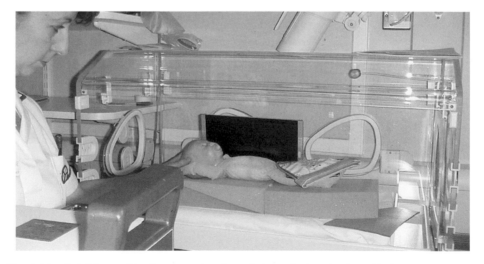

**Fig. 6.30** A doll is used to demonstrate a lateral abdominal projection with the neonate in the supine decubitus position.

to allow visualisation of the la teral abdominal walls and the legs should be extended at the hips to prevent superimposition over the lower abdomen.

## Inverted lateral rectum

The inverted lateral projection for rectal atresia should only be undertaken when the neonate is at least 18 hours old so that air will have had opportunity to travel to the site of obstruction. The neonate should be placed in an inverted prone position over a foam pad or small pillow for at least 10 minutes prior to exposure to allow air to rise to the proximal site of obstruction (Fig. 6.31). A horizontal beam lateral projection of the pelvis is taken with the central ray centred to the greater trochanter. An opaque marker may be placed on the anal dimple to show the distal site of the obstruction. The resultant radiograph should include the whole of the sacrum (Fig. 6.32).

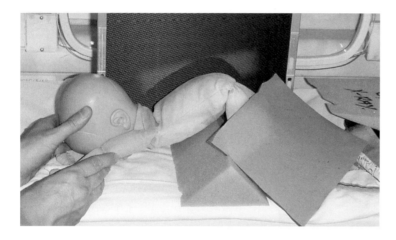

**Fig. 6.31** A doll is used to demonstrate positioning for an inverted lateral rectum for imperforate anus.

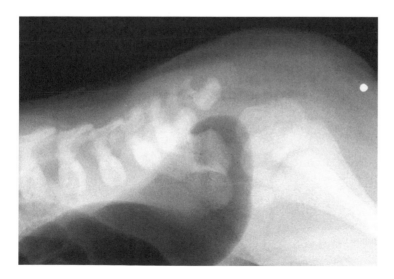

**Fig. 6.32** Horizontal beam lateral rectum for imperforate anus. Note the lead shot to indicate the anus.

**Box 6.6**   Exposure factors – neonatal abdominal radiography (adapted from the European Guidelines on Quality Criteria for Diagnostic Radiographic Images in Paediatrics[16]).

| | |
|---|---|
| Nominal focal spot value: | 0.6 mm |
| Focus-to-film distance (FFD): | 100 cm |
| Kilovoltage: | 65–85 kV |
| Exposure time: | < 20 ms |
| Film-screen system: | nominal speed class 400–800 |
| Additional filtration: | up to 1 mm Al + 0.1 or 0.2 mm Cu (or equivalent) |
| Anti-scatter grid: | none |

### Exposure factors

The European Guidelines on Quality Criteria for Diagnostic Radiographic Images in Paediatrics[16] recommends the use of a kilovoltage in the range 65–85 kV (Box 6.6). This is a relatively high kV technique that results in relatively low radiographic contrast in the image, but it also has the advantages of reducing patient dose and permitting the use of shorter exposure times. Patient dose may also be further reduced through the use of a fast film screen combination. An exposure time of less than 20 ms will reduce the risk of recorded movement unsharpness due to respiration and bowel peristalsis. The use of an automatic exposure control or grid is not recommended due to the small abdominal size and difficulties in positioning a chamber accurately to an appropriate dominant area. The recommended focus-to-film distance is 100–115 cm with additional tube filtration of up to 1 mm aluminium + 0.1 or 0.2 mm copper. This filtration gives a relatively 'hard' beam of x-rays that reduces the quantity of low energy photons in the beam and therefore reduces the dose to the patient.

The image criteria for assessing the technical quality of an abdominal radiograph is discussed in Chapter 5.

## Summary

This chapter has aimed to highlight some of the more common indications and radiographic examinations undertaken during the neonatal period and to raise the radiographer's awareness of the organisation of neonatal units and the role of the radiographer within the multiprofessional team. It is important that any radiographer undertaking neonatal radiography is able to appreciate the operation of these units and can effectively communicate with nursing and medical staff in order to provide high-quality diagnostic images.

## References

1.   Kelnar, C.J.H., Harvey, D. and Simpson, C. (1995) *The Sick Newborn Baby*, 3rd edn. Baillière Tindall, London.

2.  Rennie, J.M. and Roberton, N.R.C. (1999) *Textbook of Neonatology*, 3rd edn. Churchill Livingstone, Edinburgh.
3.  Campbell, A.G.M. and McIntosh, N. (1998*) Forfar and Arneil's Textbook of Pediatrics*, 5th edn. Churchill Livingstone, Edinburgh.
4.  Roberton, N.R.C. (1993) *A Manual of Neonatal Intensive Care*, 3rd edn. Edward Arnold, London.
5.  American Academy of Pediatrics (1997) Noise: A hazard for the fetus and newborn [Policy Statement]. *Pediatrics* **100** (4) 724–27.
6.  Erkonen, W.E. (ed.) (1998) *Radiology 101: The Basics and Fundamentals of Imaging*. Lippincott-Raven, Philadelphia.
7.  Weissleder, R. and Wittenberg, J. (1994) *Primer of Diagnostic Imaging*. Mosby, London.
8.  Behram, R.E. and Kliegman, R.M. (1994) *Essentials of Pediatrics*, 2nd edn. WB Saunders Company, London.
9.  Grainger, R.G., Allison, D.J., Adam, A. and Dixon, A.K. (2001) *Grainger and Allison's Diagnostic Radiology – A Textbook of Medical Imaging*, 4th edn. Churchill Livingstone, London.
10.  Juhl, J.H., Crummy, A.B. and Kuhlman, J.E. (1998) *Essentials of Radiologic Imaging*, 7th edn. Lippincott-Raven, New York.
11.  Halliday, H.L., McClure, B.G. and Reid, M. (1998) *Handbook of Neonatal Intensive Care*, 4th edn. WB Saunders Company, London.
12.  Bates, J.A. (1999) *Abdominal Ultrasound*. Churchill Livingstone, Edinburgh.
13.  Blickman, J.G. (1994) *Pediatric Radiology: The Requisites*. Mosby, London.
14.  Pritzker School of Medicine Paediatric Clerkship (2000–01) Abdominal masses in neonates. [Online] Feb 2002
(http://pedclerk.bsd.uchicago.edu/abdominalInNeonates.html).
15.  Sutton, D. (ed.) (1998) *A Textbook of Radiology and Imaging*, 6th edn. Churchill Livingstone, London.
16.  Kohn, M.M., Moores, B.M., Schibilla, H. *et al.* (eds) (1996) *European Guidelines on Quality Criteria for Diagnostic Radiographic Images in Paediatrics* (EUR 16261 EN). Office for Official Publications of the European Communities, Luxembourg.
17.  Meerstadt, P.W.D. and Gyll, C. (1994) *Manual of Neonatal Emergency X-ray Interpretation*. WB Saunders Company Ltd, London.

*Further reading*

Balfour-Lynn, I.M. and Valman, H.B. (1993) *Practical Management of the Newborn*, 5th edn. Blackwell Scientific Publications, Oxford.

# Chapter 7
# Skeletal trauma

Paediatric patients account for approximately 30% of casualty attendances in the UK[1] and many of these children are referred for skeletal radiography to confirm or exclude a fracture. Skeletal fractures constitute between 10 and 25% of all childhood injuries and it is therefore essential that radiographers have a working knowledge of the trauma mechanisms and injury patterns appropriate to children in order to assist them in the appropriate imaging and identification of paediatric trauma. This chapter aims to discuss common skeletal injuries in children and aspects of radiographic pattern recognition in order to enable the radiographer to more thoroughly understand this field.

## Children's fractures

Skeletal fractures occur as a result of tensile, compressive or shearing forces. These forces can work in isolation or in combination to create specific and identifiable fracture patterns (Figs 7.1 and 7.2).

Children's bones are different to mature adult bones in that they are less well calcified, are more porous and have greater elasticity and flexibility. As a result, the fracture patterns seen are different to those seen in adults and, with the exception of high-energy trauma incidents such as road traffic accidents, childhood injuries tend to be of the limbs rather than the axial skeleton (Box 7.1 and Figs 7.3–7.7).

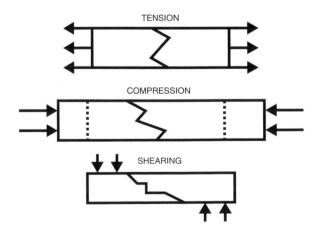

**Fig. 7.1** Forces that may cause skeletal fractures.

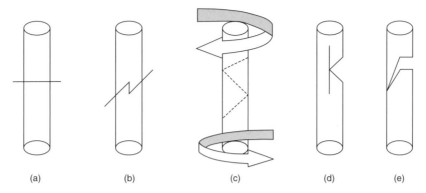

**Fig. 7.2** Fracture types and their associated causative forces. (a) Transverse fracture (tensile force). (b) Oblique fracture (compressive force). (c) Spiral fracture (rotational force). (d) Incomplete fracture (angulation with compression). (e) Transverse + oblique fracture (tensile + compressive forces).

True joint dislocations rarely occur as a result of trauma in children. Instead, epiphyseal displacement results as the injury force is focused on the physeal region. Injuries around the physis are common in children as the physis is the main point of weakness in children's long bones. The ligaments surrounding the joint are often stronger than the bone and, therefore, unlike the adult, a child is more likely to suffer fractures, including those into the physis, than ligamentous injuries and joint dislocations.

To ensure that paediatric injuries are accurately diagnosed, a comprehensive system of radiographic assessment should be implemented and clues to assist in the recognition of trauma will be discussed within this chapter. However, it should be noted that, as with adults, occult trauma may not be identified on the initial radiographs and further imaging should be considered if the patient's clinical symptoms fail to resolve within 7–10 days.

**Box 7.1** Common childhood fractures.

*Greenstick fracture*:   Bending and angulation forces tense the convex and compress the concave sides of the bone causing an incomplete transverse fracture on the convex side extending to the bone centre and a buckling deformity on the concave side.

*Torus fracture*:   A cortical deformity caused by compression and is usually metaphyseal in location.

*Lead pipe fracture*:   An incomplete transverse fracture of one cortex with an associated buckling of the opposite side. The lead pipe fracture is generally found in the metaphysis.

*Plastic bowing fracture*:   Occurs as a result of deformation forces exceeding the elastic strain capability of the bone. Although an obvious fracture may not be generated, the bone appears bowed (bent) throughout its length.

*Toddler's fracture*:   A non-displaced oblique fracture, usually of the tibial shaft, that typically is only seen on one radiographic projection. It occurs in children between the ages of 1 and 3 years and is thought to be a result of the torsional forces that occur when the young child grips the floor with their toes when learning to walk.

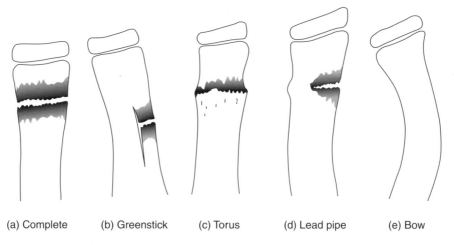

(a) Complete     (b) Greenstick     (c) Torus     (d) Lead pipe     (e) Bow

**Fig. 7.3**   Common fracture patterns in children.

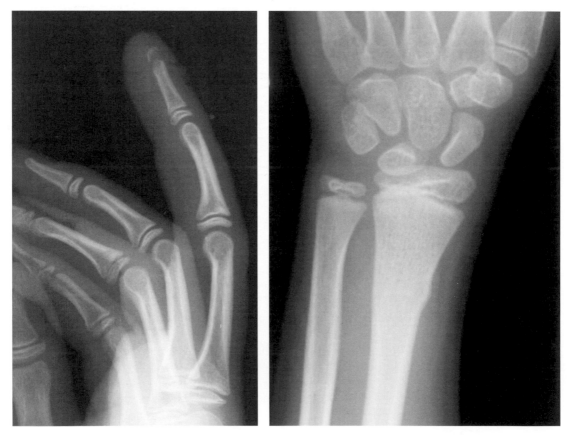

**Fig. 7.4**   Complete fracture of distal phalanx.     **Fig. 7.5**   Torus fracture of distal radius.

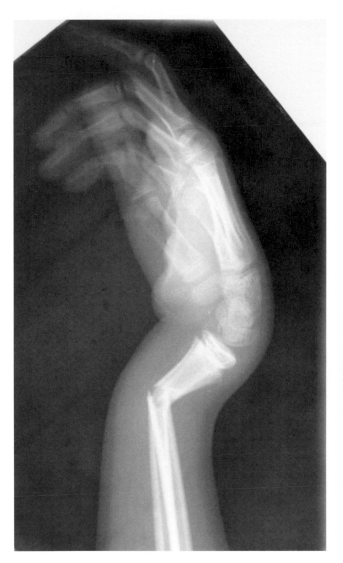

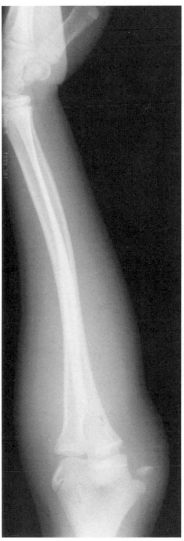

**Fig. 7.6** Greenstick fracture of radius and ulna.

**Fig. 7.7** Plastic bowing forearm fracture. Note the associated avulsion of the medial epicondyle of the humerus.

## The epiphyses

The epiphyses are the secondary ossification centres related to bone growth. Epiphyseal injuries result from shearing forces directed through the epiphyseal plate, avulsive forces focused through the ligamentous and joint capsular attachments and vertical forces directed to the centre of the epiphysis. Accurate identification of an epiphyseal injury is essential because of its association with bone growth disturbances and possible failure of the bone to form the correct shape or joint relationships[2].

**Table 7.1**  Percentage bone growth at appendicular epiphyses.

| Bone | Physeal growth |
| --- | --- |
| Humerus | Proximal = 80% |
| | Distal = 20% |
| Radius | Proximal = 25% |
| | Distal = 75% |
| Ulna | Proximal = 20% |
| | Distal = 80% |
| Femur | Proximal = 30% |
| | Distal = 70% |
| Tibia | Proximal = 55% |
| | Distal = 45% |

Most epiphyseal injuries occur between the ages of 10 and 16 years (with the exception of the distal humeral epiphysis where most injuries are noted in children under 10 years of age). The likelihood of an epiphyseal injury adversely affecting bone growth is dependent upon its type and site, as the rate of physeal growth is not consistent within the body (Table 7.1). The most commonly used system for classifying physeal fractures is the Salter-Harris classification system (Table 7.2 and Figs 7.8–7.12).

The management of physeal injuries varies from simple immobilisation to complex surgical procedures. Essentially, Salter-Harris type I and type II injuries will retain an intact epiphysis and can be treated by closed immobilisation following minimal reduction. Salter-Harris type III and type IV injuries may require surgical intervention as the epiphyseal fragments are separate and mobile. Salter-Harris type V injuries cannot be treated directly as these injuries result from physeal compression and the subsequent closure of the growth plate prevents further growth. In these patients, regular growth assessment will be necessary to evaluate any limb length discrepancy.

# Upper limb injuries

## The clavicle

The fracture and dislocation of the clavicle is a frequent childhood shoulder injury, particularly in children under 10 years of age. The injury pattern is typically a greenstick fracture of the middle third of the clavicle with no associated ligamentous damage (Fig. 7.13). Occasionally, in 5% of injuries, a fracture of the outer third of the clavicle may be seen and any displacement at this site is suggestive of coracoclavicular ligamentous damage. The coracoclavicular and acromioclavicular ligaments hold the clavicle in position and damage to these ligaments can result in clavicular subluxation or dislocation[2] (Box 7.2).

**Table 7.2**   The Salter-Harris classification system.

| Salter-Harris type | Features | Diagram |
|---|---|---|
| I | Separation of the metaphysis and epiphysis which is seen radiographically as misalignment or widening of the physis<br><br>Accounts for 6–8% of injuries and is most commonly seen in children under 5 years of age | |
| II | Separation of physis (with or without misalignment) plus a metaphyseal fracture<br><br>Commonest fracture pattern and accounts for 70% of injuries<br><br>Most frequently seen in distal radius injuries and in children over 8 years of age | |
| III | An intra-articular fracture through the epiphysis which results in a separated epiphyseal fragment<br><br>Accounts for 7% of injuries and is commonly seen in the distal femoral and tibial epiphyses | |
| IV | An intra-articular fracture through the epiphysis, physeal plate and metaphysis<br><br>Accounts for approximately 12% of injuries and is most frequently seen in the lateral condyle of the humerus | |
| V | Compression of the physis which has serious prognostic consequences<br><br>This is the most serious physeal injury and accounts for 0.5% of injuries. It is most commonly seen in the distal tibia and femur but can be difficult to identify, particularly after fusion across the physis has begun in adolescence | |

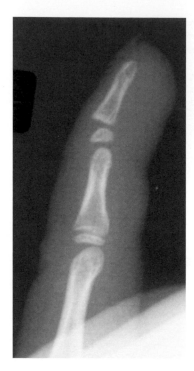

**Fig. 7.8**   Salter-Harris type I injury of the distal phalanx.

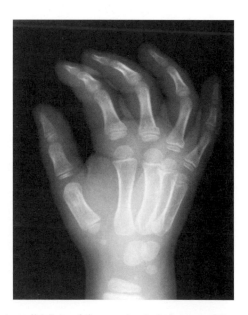

**Fig. 7.9**   Salter-Harris type II injury of the proximal phalanges of the second, third and fourth fingers.

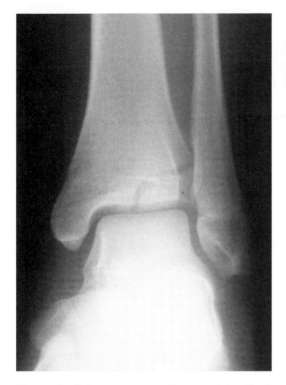

**Fig. 7.10** Salter-Harris type III injury of the distal tibia.

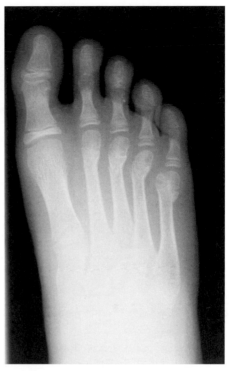

**Fig. 7.11** Salter-Harris type IV injury of the fifth metatarsal head.

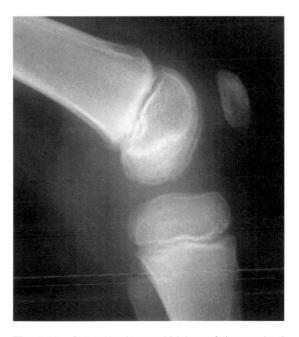

**Fig. 7.12** Salter-Harris type V injury of the proximal tibia posteriorly.

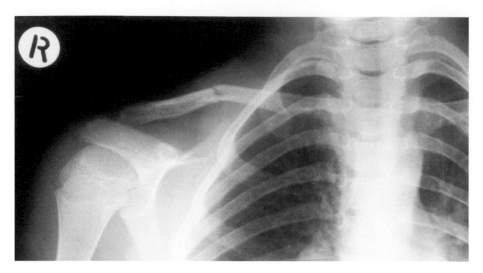

**Fig. 7.13**   Fracture of the middle third of the clavicle.

**Box 7.2**   Classification of acromioclavicular and coracoclavicular ligament disruption.

*Type 1*:   Spraining of the acromioclavicular ligaments with no movement of the clavicle.

*Type 2*:   Tearing of the acromioclavicular ligaments with coracoclavicular ligaments remaining intact. Minimal malalignment may be seen with displacement of the acromioclavicular joint of up to half the thickness of the clavicle.

*Type 3*:   Tearing of both the acromioclavicular and the coracoclavicular ligaments with possible associated avulsion of the coracoid process. The acromioclavicular joint is widened and the clavicle is seen above the level of the acromion process.

## The scapula

The scapula is rarely fractured owing to its thick covering of muscles and therefore significant force is necessary to cause injury (e.g. direct blows to the shoulder may cause scapular neck fractures or a vertically directed force may fracture the acromion). The secondary ossification centres on the lateral aspect of the acromion can cause confusion and it is important to remember that they do not appear until between the ages of 15 and 18 years and can be fragmented in appearance.

## The glenohumeral joint

Dislocation at the glenohumeral joint is rare in children as the proximal humeral growth plate forms a natural line of weakness and will transmit any force to generate a Salter-Harris type injury. However, if a true dislocation does occur, it is likely to be in an anterior direction (97% of cases) following a fall on an outstretched hand.

## The proximal humerus

Proximal humerus injuries tend to be Salter-Harris type I injuries in infants and Salter-Harris type II injuries in older children (Figs 7.14 and 7.15). Humeral shaft fractures will commonly occur following direct trauma and may have an associated open wound whereas transverse, oblique and spiral fractures are generated by indirect forces. Up to 25% of humeral shaft fractures will have an associated elbow, shoulder or clavicular injury and, therefore, it is essential that the whole of the humerus is imaged including the elbow and shoulder joints.

## The elbow

The elbow is a complicated joint both to adequately image and to interpret and, as a result, several lines and systems of review have evolved to assist in the accurate diagnosis of elbow trauma. The first system to be considered here is known as CRITOL.

The elbow has six secondary ossification centres that ossify in sequence and these can be remembered as the mnemonic CRITOL (Fig. 7.16). The order of ossification can assist the radiographer in identifying true trauma from normal ossification appearances. For example, if trochlear ossification is apparent but the radial head has not yet ossified then it is likely that the appearances are related to trauma rather than normal elbow ossification. In addition, the age at which the secondary centres of the elbow ossify can also help in the diagnosis of subtle elbow trauma[3] (Box 7.3).

Other useful review tools are the anterior humeral line and the radiocapitellar line (Fig. 7.17). The anterior humeral line should be drawn along the anterior humeral cortex on the lateral elbow projection and should pass through the anterior to the middle third of the capitellum in a normal elbow (Fig. 7.18). However, care must be taken as this line is only useful if the elbow is imaged in a truly lateral position. In contrast, the radiocapitellar line can be successfully applied to all elbow projections and it should be drawn through the middle of the proximal radial shaft to intersect with the centre of the capitellum in the normal elbow (Fig. 7.17). Failure of the radiocapitellar line to intersect with the capitellum on any one projection suggests dislocation or subluxation at the radiocapitellar joint.

Elevated fat pads, seen on the lateral elbow projection, are a good indication that an intercapsular fracture is present, even if the fracture cannot be identified

**Box 7.3** Appearance of secondary ossification centres of the elbow.

| | |
|---|---|
| **C**apitellum | 2 months–2 years |
| **R**adial head | 3–6 years |
| **I**nternal (medial) epicondyle | 4–7 years |
| **T**rochlea | 8–10 years |
| **O**lecranon | 8–10 years |
| **L**ateral epicondyle | 10–13 years |

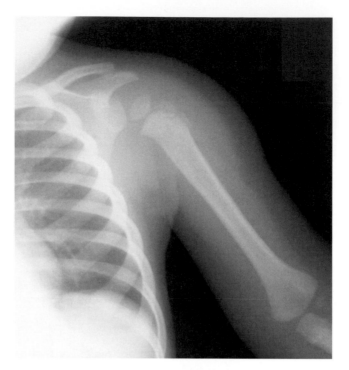

**Fig. 7.14**   Salter-Harris type II injury of the proximal humerus.

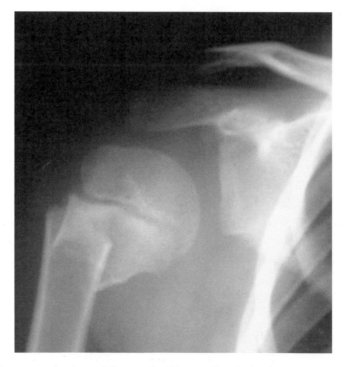

**Fig. 7.15**   Transverse fracture of the proximal humeral metaphysis.

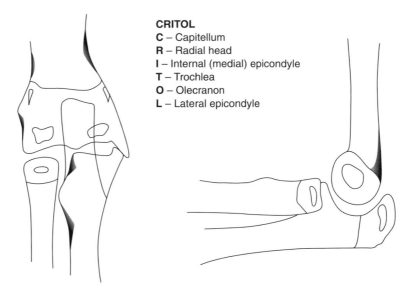

**Fig. 7.16**   The secondary ossification centres of the elbow.

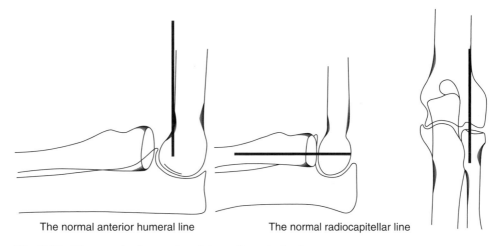

The normal anterior humeral line            The normal radiocapitellar line

**Fig. 7.17**   The anterior humeral and the radiocapitellar lines.

on the initial radiograph[4]. The anterior fat pad, which sits in the shallow coronoid fossa of the humerus, can be seen on most lateral elbow projections but its position is more markedly raised following trauma (the sail sign). The posterior fat pad sits in the deeper olecranon fossa and is rarely seen unless elevated as a consequence of trauma and is therefore a more significant finding (Fig. 7.19).

## Supracondylar fracture

The supracondylar fracture accounts for approximately 60% of all elbow injuries in children[5]. It typically results from a fall on an outstretched hand while the

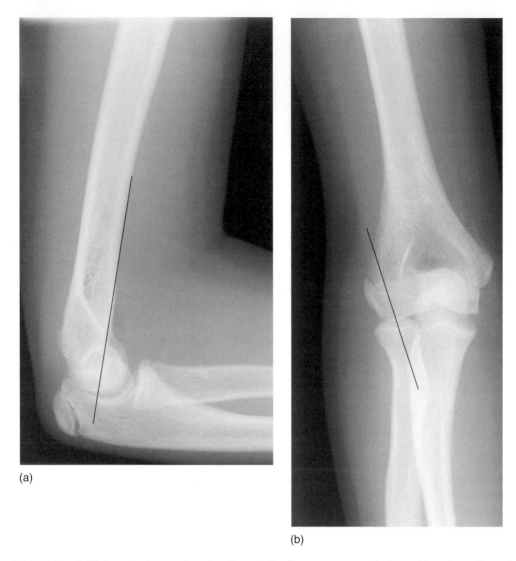

(a)

(b)

**Fig. 7.18**   (a) and (b) Anterior humeral and radiocapitellar lines on a normal elbow. Note the radiocapitellar line is drawn through the proximal radial shaft.

elbow is held in extension and most commonly occurs between the ages of 4 and 8 years (Fig. 7.20). A subtle supracondylar fracture line may not be visible on the antero-posterior projection of the elbow. However, the lateral projection will generally show anterior and posterior fat pad displacement and posterior movement of the humeral condyles relative to the humeral shaft when assessed using the anterior humeral line (Fig. 7.21).

### Condyles

Isolated lateral humeral condyle fractures account for up to 20% of all paediatric elbow injuries and frequently result from a fall on an outstretched hand (Fig.

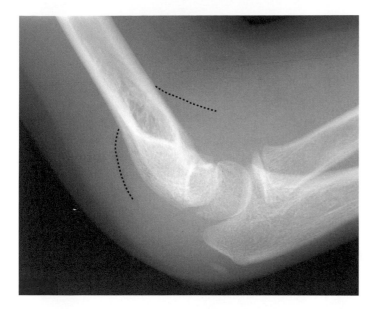

**Fig. 7.19**   Raised anterior and posterior fat pads (dashed lines).

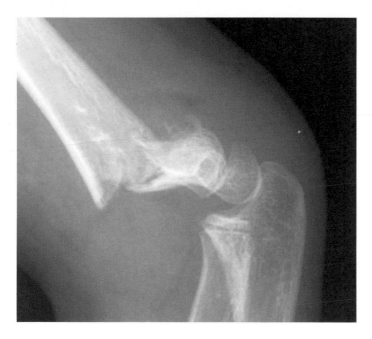

**Fig. 7.20**   Severe supracondylar fracture.

7.22). They are generally reported as Salter-Harris type III or type IV injuries involving the capitellum and are most commonly seen in children between the ages of 5 and 10 years. Identification of this injury is important as the fracture fragment can be pulled postero-inferiorly and result in valgus deformity, ulnar nerve palsy and premature physeal fusion unless adequate reduction is achieved[6]. In contrast, isolated medial humeral condyle fractures are rare and usually present as a Salter-Harris type IV injury.

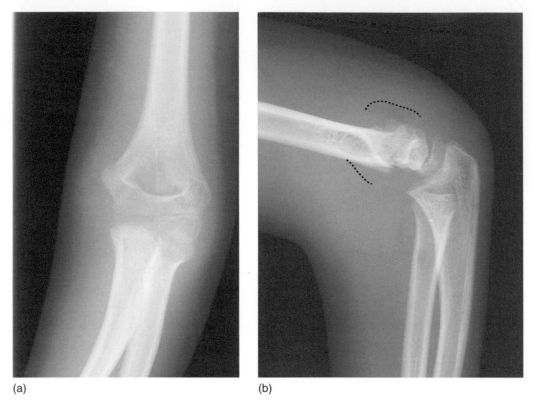

(a)

(b)

**Fig. 7.21** (a) and (b) Subtle supracondylar fracture. Note that although a fracture line is difficult to identify on the antero-posterior projection (a), raised fat pads (dashed lines) and posteriorly displaced humeral condyles on the lateral projection (b) indicate the presence of a supracondylar fracture.

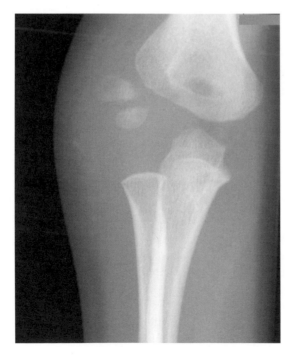

**Fig. 7.22** Fracture of the lateral humeral condyle with associated displacement of the capitellum. Note the radiocapitellar line is maintained.

## *Epicondyles*

Avulsion of the medial epicondyle accounts for approximately 10% of all paediatric elbow injuries and is typically seen between the ages of 7 and 15 years.
The mechanism of injury is commonly a fall on an outstretched hand resulting
in severe valgus elbow strain. The avulsed medial epicondyle will generally
move inferiorly and may become trapped within the elbow joint space where it
can be confused with the trochlear ossification centre. As the epicondyle may lie
outside the joint capsule, this injury will not necessarily have an associated effusion and elevated fat pads. The most useful evaluation tool to ensure that this
injury is not missed is therefore the CRITOL mnemonic (Fig. 7.23).

## *Proximal radius*

Although common in adults, radial head injuries are rare in children as
ossification of the radial head is not complete until approximately 10 years
of age. Instead, Salter-Harris type II fractures of the radial neck tend to occur
and these injuries are best demonstrated on the lateral elbow projection
(Fig. 7.24).

## *Proximal ulna*

Fractures of the proximal ulna tend to involve the olecranon process (Fig. 7.25),
but care should be taken as the olecranon ossification centre can often appear
fragmented and should not be confused with a fracture. Olecranon fractures
occur following a fall on an outstretched hand or as a result of a direct blow
to the elbow and are frequently associated with proximal radius fractures
(Fig. 7.26). Separation of the fracture fragments can occur on contraction of the
triceps muscle if the fracture is distal to the site of the triceps muscle insertion
(Fig. 7.27).

## *Elbow dislocations*

Although true joint dislocations are rare in children, a dislocation at the elbow
may occur and typically results in posterior movement of the radius and ulna
relative to the humerus[7] (Fig. 7.28). The mechanism of injury is usually a fall on
an outstretched hand and an associated fracture of the coronoid process, as a
result of impaction against the trochlea, may be seen. Occasionally, following
complex trauma, more unusual dislocations occur and radiographers should be
wary of the rare true medial or lateral dislocation which can appear normal on
the lateral elbow projection. Separation of the entire distal humeral epiphysis in
very young children may be confused with a joint dislocation. However, maintenance of the normal radiocapitellar relationship differentiates this injury from
a true dislocation.

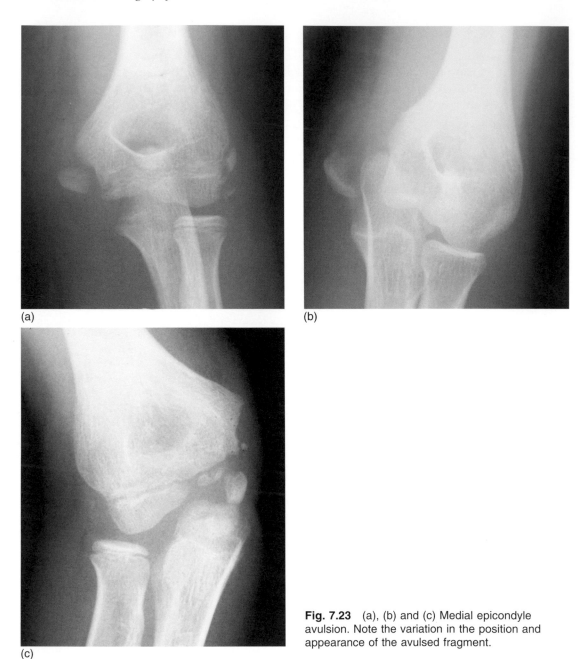

(a)

(b)

(c)

**Fig. 7.23**   (a), (b) and (c) Medial epicondyle avulsion. Note the variation in the position and appearance of the avulsed fragment.

## The forearm

Radial and ulnar mid-shaft fractures rarely occur in isolation and the radiographer should look carefully for an associated injury to the other forearm bone, or disruption at the elbow or wrist joint. It is not uncommon for fractures of both the radius and ulna to occur at the same level following direct trauma (Fig. 7.29). Alternatively, a fracture of one bone may be associated with a plastic bowing

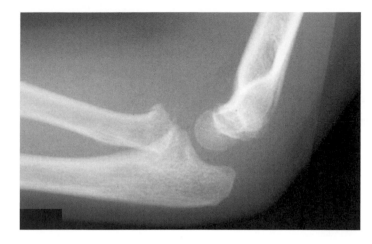

**Fig. 7.24** Salter-Harris type II fracture of the proximal radius.

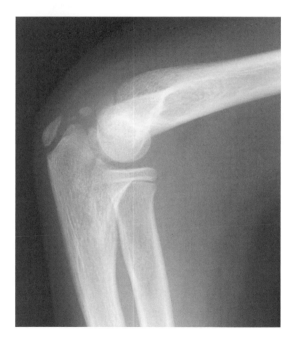

**Fig. 7.25** Subtle isolated intra-articular fracture of the proximal ulna.

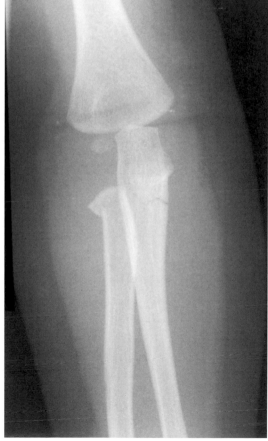

**Fig. 7.26** Proximal ulnar and radius fractures.

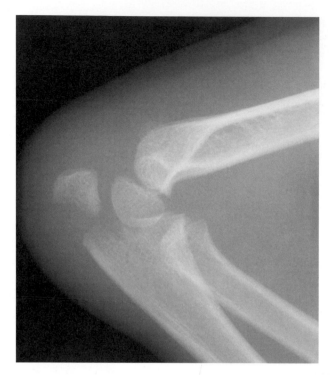

**Fig. 7.27**   Separation of olecranon fracture fragments following contraction of the triceps muscle.

deformity of the other. Monteggia-type lesions, consisting of a mid-shaft ulna fracture with associated anterior radial head dislocation, are seen in children in many forms[2] and it is essential that forearm radiographs include both wrist and elbow joints to allow the accurate assessment of bony alignment and reveal any associated joint injuries.

## The wrist

The most common childhood skeletal injury is the distal radius fracture. In young children, these are typically torus, greenstick or complete in nature and are predominantly found in the metaphyseal region[8,9]. In older children, fractures of the distal radius typically involve the epiphyseal plate and are classified using the Salter-Harris classification system (Table 7.2 and Figs 7.30 and 7.31).

Injuries to the carpal bones are rare in children. A fracture of the scaphoid bone may be seen in children over the age of 10 years but this will typically occur at the distal pole or tubercle rather than at the scaphoid waist and therefore avascular problems are rarely encountered. However, a creeping sclerosis or porosity is suggestive of avascular necrosis and in these cases further imaging (MRI or scintigraphy) is advocated in order to confirm the diagnosis.

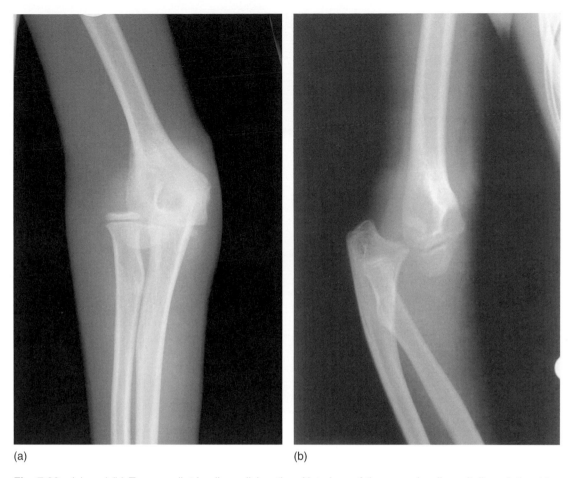

(a)                                    (b)

**Fig. 7.28**   (a) and (b) True paediatric elbow dislocation. Note loss of the normal radiocapitellar relationship.

## The hand

The hand is covered by a minimum of soft tissue and is relatively delicate. As a result, crushing injuries to the hand frequently cause comminution, soft tissue damage and ligamentous tears. Although it has been suggested that hand injuries in children over 4 years of age occur predominantly in males[10], it is not until they enter adolescence that boys are particularly associated with a specific injury – the 'punch' fracture[11,12] (Figs 7.32 and 7.33). This injury, which results in a fracture to the neck or shaft of the fifth metacarpal with associated palmar angulation of the distal fragment, may be complicated by osteomyelitis if a bite injury at the fracture site has also been sustained.

A fracture of the base of the first metacarpal (Bennett's fracture) is also frequently seen in children and is typically classified as a Salter-Harris type II injury with or without epiphyseal displacement.

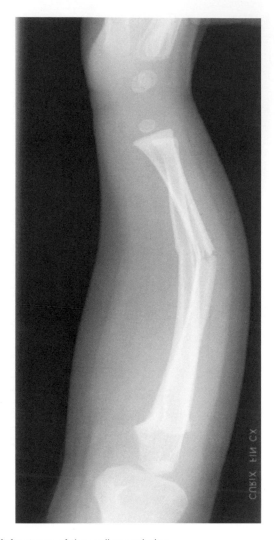

**Fig. 7.29**    Mid-shaft fractures of the radius and ulna.

Finger injuries in young children tend to result from crushing mechanisms (e.g. car doors), while in older children sporting activities may result in forced flexion and extension finger injuries (Fig. 7.34).

# Lower limb injuries

### The hip

Femoral neck fractures are rarely found in children unless they have been involved in a road traffic accident or fallen from a considerable height. Instead, as with upper limb trauma, injury forces tend to focus upon the epiphyseal

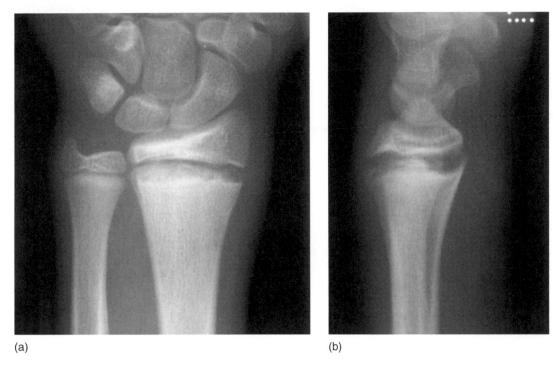

(a)                                                     (b)

**Fig. 7.30** (a) and (b) Widening of the distal radial physis as a result of repetitive strain in a young athlete. May be classified as a Salter-Harris type I injury.

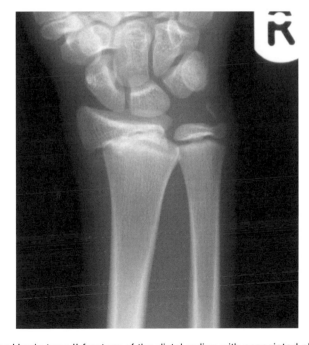

**Fig. 7.31** Salter-Harris type II fracture of the distal radius with associated slipped epiphysis.

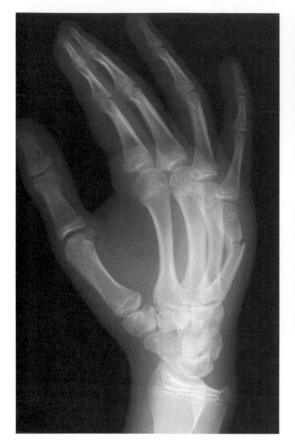

**Fig. 7.32**   Typical appearances of a 'punch' injury.

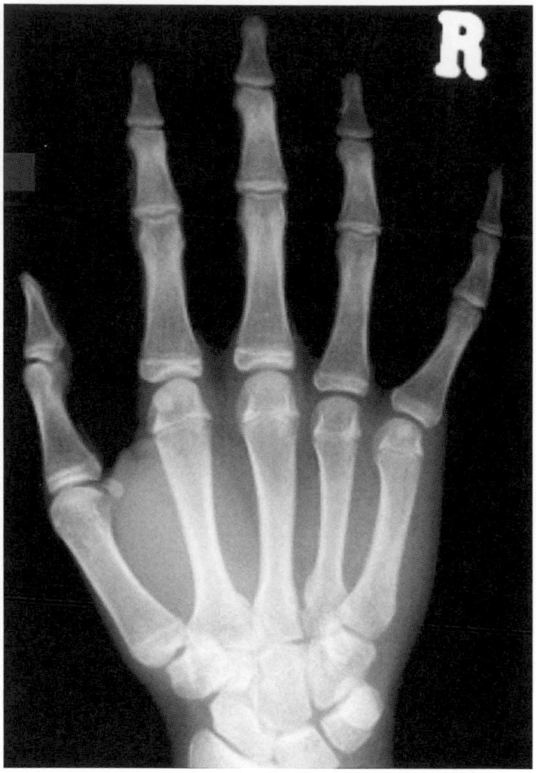

**Fig. 7.33**   An unusual vertical fracture of the distal shaft of the fifth metacarpal caused by a punching injury.

region. The femoral capital epiphysis begins to ossify between 3 and 6 months of age, calcifying in a centrifugal pattern. The epiphysis reaches completion by 8 years of age and fuses with the femoral neck between the ages of 16 and 19 years. The lesser trochanter does not commence ossification until approximately 8 years but fusion once again occurs between the ages of 16 and 19 years. In infants, the continuity of cartilage between the greater trochanter and the femoral head ensures that the hip performs as a single epiphyseal unit. As a result, trauma to the infant hip typically results in a Salter-Harris type I injury.

### Femoral shaft injuries

Direct trauma is the main cause of femoral shaft fractures and injury patterns include the complete, oblique or transverse fracture and, in the very young child, the spiral fracture. Additional and associated femoral injuries are noted in the same limb in around one third of cases whilst almost a half show associated injuries elsewhere in the body. Healing of a femoral fracture is generally good,

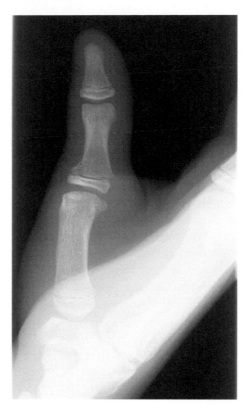

**Fig. 7.34** Salter-Harris type II fracture of the proximal phalanx of the thumb.

particularly in the very young child, and abundant callus formation can be seen. However, an unfortunate sequelae of a femoral fracture may be limb length discrepancy which, if not corrected, can lead to pelvic tilting and spinal scoliosis.

### Distal femoral injuries

Injuries to the distal femoral metaphysis will generally involve the physeal plate and can be classified according to the Salter-Harris classification system (typically Salter-Harris type I or type II injuries). Epiphyseal injuries tend to be of a Salter-Harris type IV classification with a T- or Y-shaped deformity through the epiphysis being seen communicating with the joint. Damage to the distal femoral epiphysis is important as 70% of femoral growth occurs here and therefore the consequences of any growth disturbance can be serious (Table 7.1).

### The knee

The knee is the largest joint in the body and is susceptible to damage from play and sporting activities such as running and jumping. Radiographic assessment of the knee following trauma can be problematic and it is important that the soft tissues are clearly visible. A horizontal beam lateral projection should be undertaken routinely following trauma to demonstrate any effusion or lipo-haemarthrosis within the suprapatellar bursa (Fig. 7.35).

## The patella

The patella is the largest sesamoid bone in the body and ossification commences between 2 and 6 years of age. As a result, the patella is rarely injured until mid adolescence. A normal variation in patella ossification, which can be easily confused for a patella fracture, is the bipartite patella where a smooth, rounded and apparently extra piece of bone is seen on the supero-lateral border of the patella. Other normal variants include the multipartite patella and the appearance of the patella as a vestigial structure as a result of speckled ossification. An apophysis may also be noted on the anterior surface of the patella. Where patella fractures do occur in the older adolescent, their appearances mimic those found in the adult with open lesions, comminution and transverse fractures being common. Separation of the fracture fragments may also be seen as a result of the quadriceps tendon and patellar ligament pulling in opposite directions.

## The tibia and fibula

Ossification of the proximal tibial epiphysis is noted at approximately 3 months of age whereas ossification of the proximal fibular epiphysis is not seen until 2 to 4 years of age. Both growth plates fuse at approximately 15 years.

Proximal tibial injuries are relatively rare and tend to present as Salter-Harris type II injuries in young adults. In children between the ages of 8 and 15 years, a fall from a bicycle with the knee in flexion can result in a fracture of the inter-condylar eminence/tibial spine, tearing of the anterior cruciate ligament or, rarely, a tibial tuberosity fracture[13] (Fig. 7.36). In contrast, a hyperextension injury

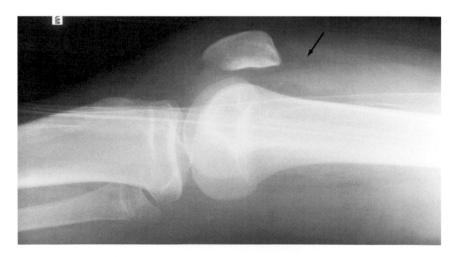

**Fig. 7.35** Lipohaemarthrosis (arrow points to position of fatty tissue).

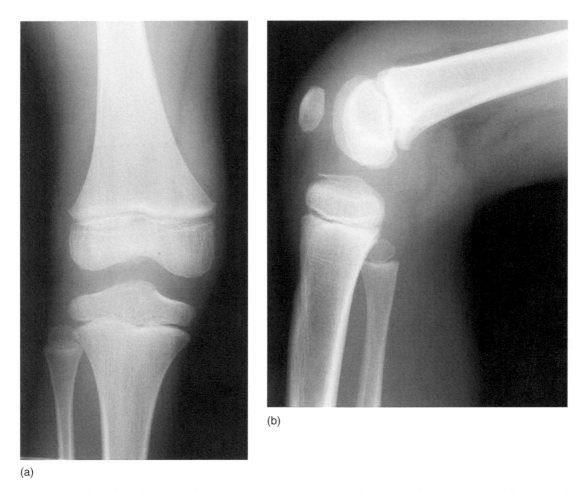

(b)

(a)

**Fig. 7.36** (a) and (b) Fracture of the intercondylar eminence at the site of the anterior cruciate ligament attachment.

may result in the avulsion of the posterior cruciate ligament and radiographs should be carefully scrutinised for associated bony fragments. As the injury forces are focused at the proximal tibial epiphysis, a true knee dislocation is rare in the immature skeleton. However, once physeal fusion has occurred, dislocations may be seen and these can be associated with soft tissue and nerve or vascular damage.

Proximal tibial metaphyseal fractures are seen between the ages of 3 and 6 years and all Salter-Harris fracture patterns are seen. Occasionally, an associated greenstick fracture of the fibula is also noted. Proximal fibular fractures are rarely seen in isolation and, if not directly associated with a proximal tibial fracture, result from the transmission of forces from the ankle joint following lateral rotation of the ankle. In these circumstances the injury is typically a spiral fracture of the fibular neck and, once again, associated nerve or vascular damage may occur.

## The toddler's fracture

The toddler's fracture is probably the most well-known isolated mid-shaft fracture of the tibia and is typically seen between the ages of 1 and 3 years (Fig. 7.37). Clinical presentation is often the acute onset of a limp with no specific cause. Radiographically, the toddler's fracture is seen as a spiral fracture of the tibial shaft with minimal displacement and is commonly only seen on one projection. An associated greenstick fibular fracture or dislocation of the proximal tibiofibular joint may also occur as a result of disruption to the tibiofibular ring. Other

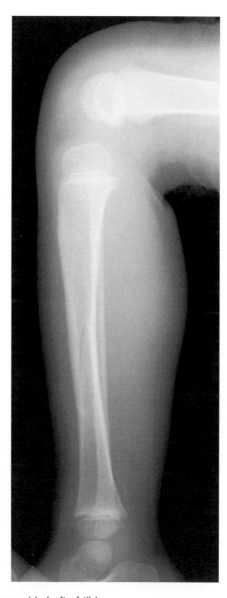

**Fig. 7.37**  Toddler fracture mid-shaft of tibia.

documented 'toddler' injuries that should be considered when a young child presents with an acute limp are a spiral fracture of the femur or a fracture of the calcaneus, patella, cuboid or pubic rami[14].

## Stress fracture

Stress fractures result from repeated exercise and strain and are therefore usually seen in young athletes. A common site of stress fractures is the proximal tibia where radiographic examination may demonstrate a sclerotic band or dense cortical thickening (Fig. 7.38). However, diagnosis using plain film radiography may not be possible for acute conditions and, in these cases, the use of alternative imaging modalities (e.g. scintigraphy or MRI) may be appropriate.

## The ankle

The ankle mortise is formed by the distal tibia centrally and medially, the distal fibular laterally and the talar dome inferiorly. The ankle is essentially a hinge

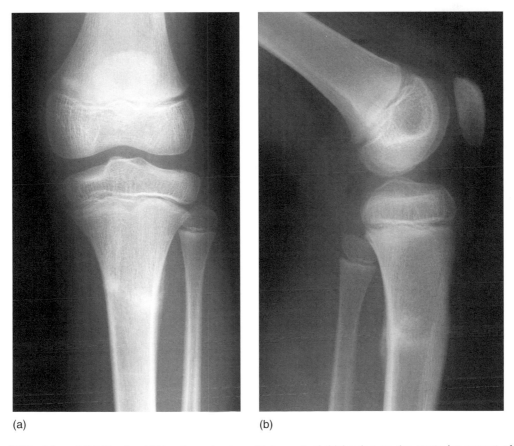

(a)                              (b)

**Fig. 7.38**   (a) and (b) Proximal tibia stress fracture. Note cortical thickening on the posterior aspect of the tibial shaft and the subtle sclerotic band through the shaft at the same level.

joint and the stability of the joint is maintained by the ligamentous structures surrounding it (Fig. 7.39). Movement at the ankle is limited to dorsiflexion and plantar-flexion with inversion and eversion occurring at the subtalar joints. Secondary ossification centres around the ankle joint can often cause confusion as a result of normal fragmentation or persistent non-union, and radiographers should have a working knowledge of common normal variants.

Ankle trauma often occurs as a result of talar movement within the mortise and specific terminology used to describe this movement is provided in Box 7.4.

With internal and external rotation of the joint, specific ankle injuries are seen and Table 7.3 describes these and their associated injury mechanisms. Injuries related to adduction tend to result in compression of the tibial physis which can cause growth arrest and may be associated with fibular overgrowth (Figs 7.40 and 7.41). For these injuries, surgical intervention may be required. The juvenile tillaux and tri-plane fractures are ankle injuries specific to the adolescent age group and occur at the time of physeal closure. Both of these injuries require prompt, accurate diagnosis and reduction in order to prevent premature degenerative changes[15,16].

It is important to remember that the ligaments surrounding the ankle joint are much stronger than the physeal plate in children and therefore physeal fractures

**Box 7.4**   Movement about the ankle joint.

> *Abduction*:   Movement of the foot/talus away from the ankle mortise (lateral direction).
>
> *Adduction*:   Movement of the foot/talus into the ankle mortise (medial direction).
>
> *Pronation*:   A combination of eversion and abduction resulting in tilting of the foot/talus laterally to rest on its medial edge.
>
> *Supination*:   A combination of inversion and adduction resulting in tilting of the foot/talus medially to rest on its lateral border.

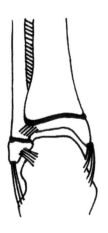 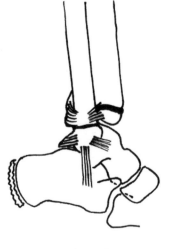

**Fig. 7.39**  Skeletal and ligamentous structures of the paediatric ankle. Note the deltoid ligament and the lateral fibulotalar and fibulocalcaneal ligaments attach to the tibial and fibular epiphyses whereas the tibiofibular ligaments attach to the tibial epiphysis and the fibular metaphysis.

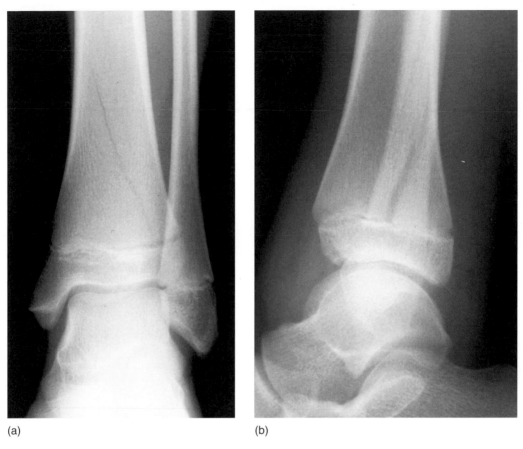

(a)                                                   (b)

**Fig. 7.40**   (a) and (b) Undisplaced Salter-Harris type II fracture of the distal tibia. Note the marked anterior capsular swelling on the lateral projection.

**Table 7.3**   Ankle injuries and their associated mechanism of trauma.

| Ankle movement | Injury description |
| --- | --- |
| Abduction with inversion and supination | Fibular avulsion via the physis. |
| Abduction with inversion and supination plus further inversion | Medial malleolar oblique fractures at the level of the tibial plafond. These are typically Salter-Harris type III or type IV injuries where the distal tibial epiphysis may shear off medially and may have an associated attached metaphyseal fragment. |
| Abduction with pronation and external rotation | The medial ligamentous structures are tensed and may result in the eventual avulsion of the medial malleolus. Lateral displacement of the tibial epiphysis allows forward and lateral talar rotation to generate a greenstick or spiral fibular fracture (Salter-Harris type II injury). |
| Supination with external rotation | The medial structures are relaxed so forcing the talus backwards and into external rotation to create an oblique distal fibular fracture. Further talar rotation will result in the distal tibial epiphysis being displaced postero-laterally with an associated posterior metaphyseal fragment. |

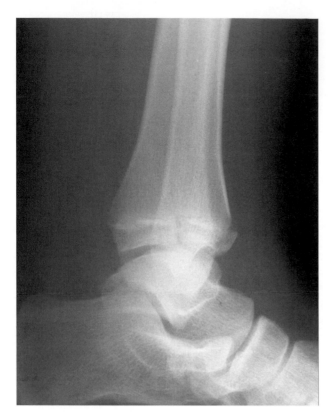

**Fig. 7.41**   Salter-Harris type III fracture. Note anterior movement of the epiphyseal fragment.

are more likely to occur than ligamentous injuries (e.g. sprains). The Ottowa ankle rules, although not specific to children, can guide the referrer in the need for radiographic assessment of ankle injuries[17] and it is important that the radiographic images are of diagnostic quality. The radiographic projections of choice are the standard mortise and lateral ankle projections. However, common errors in radiographic positioning (e.g. insufficient internal rotation and failure to place the foot in dorsiflexion) can lead to the production of suboptimal images and the misdiagnosis of subtle injuries.

### The foot

Variation in the ossification and fusion dates of the pedal epiphyses frequently leads to confusion in the identification of trauma, particularly in the infant when minimal tarsal ossification has occurred. A useful evaluation technique is therefore to remember that in feet of all ages, the talus should point to the first metatarsal and the calcaneum to the 4th or 5th metatarsal (see Chapter 8).

### The calcaneum

Calcaneal fractures are rare in pre-adolescent children and, should they occur, tend to be extra-articular and involve the tuberosity[2]. In older children, calcaneal fracture patterns mimic those of the adult; however, the associated incidence of spinal fractures is reduced. Occult 'toddler' stress fractures may present in the pre-school child but plain film examination is often negative and the use of alternative imaging modalities (scintigraphy or MRI) should be considered. Similar 'toddler' injuries may also be seen in the cuboid[18].

### The talus

Injuries to the talus must be identified owing to their propensity to develop avascular necrosis. In children, most injuries tend to involve the talar neck and a variety of fracture patterns (complete and incomplete) may be seen.

### The metatarsals

Injury to the metatarsals in children under 5 years of age tends to be confined to the 1st metatarsal whereas metatarsal injury in children over the age of 10 years is focused upon the 5th metatarsal[19]. An exception to this may be a physeal fracture at the base of the first metatarsal, usually a Salter-Harris type II injury, that may be seen in young adolescents and results from a fall from height. The apophysis of the peroneus brevis can be seen as a vertically orientated 'flake' of bone adjacent to the base of the 5th metatarsal on foot radiographs of older children (Fig. 7.42) and this should not be mistaken for a fracture at the base of the 5th metatarsal (Fig. 7.43).

### The phalanges

Fractures to the phalanges may be transverse, oblique or epiphyseal in nature and, with the exception of the distal phalanx of the great toe, have no obvious prognostic complications (Fig. 7.44). The nail bed of the great toe is attached to the physeal plate of the distal phalanx and, as a result, forced flexion injuries (i.e. stubbing the toe) will result in a Salter-Harris type I or type II injury with associated nail bed bleeding. This type of injury provides a route for the spread of infection from the nail bed to the underlying bone (osteomyelitis) and antibiotic treatment should be prescribed as a preventative measure.

## The axial skeleton

### The cervical spine

Traumatic injury to the paediatric cervical spine is rare as the neck is more flexible in children than in adults therefore allowing injury forces to spread along the length of the spine and reduce the likelihood of focal bony trauma[6]. If trauma does occur then it is likely to be concentrated in the upper cervical region (C1–C3) in children under 10 years of age. In older children, cervical spine trauma patterns mimic those seen in the adult patient. The injury mechanism for cervical

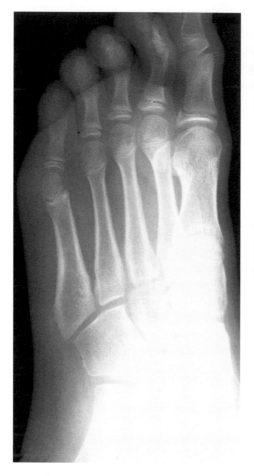

**Fig. 7.42**  Normal appearance of the peroneus brevis apophysis.

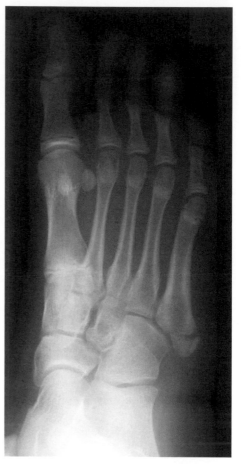

**Fig. 7.43**  A transverse intra-articular fracture at the base of the 5th metatarsal. The appearance is consistent with an inversion injury.

spine trauma in children tends to be rapid acceleration and deceleration (to create axial distraction) and may occur as a result of a road traffic accident, falls from a height, diving into the shallow end of a swimming pool or sadly, physical abuse[20–22]. Specific paediatric cervical spine injuries and their associated radiographic clues to diagnosis are described in Table 7.4.

The radiographic projections of choice for imaging the cervical spine following injury are the antero-posterior projection of C3–C7 and C1–C3, and the lateral projection from which most diagnoses will be made (Fig. 7.45). It is essential that the radiographs produced are of a high technical standard to facilitate accurate interpretation and prevent misdiagnosis. Clinical evaluation of the radiographs should include assessment of bony alignment (anterior and posterior vertebral body lines and spino-laminar line), evaluation of vertebral disc and body heights for anatomical consistency, assessment of the relationship between C1 and C2

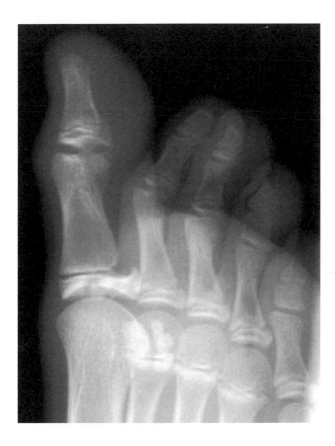

**Fig. 7.44**   Salter-Harris type III injury to the proximal epiphysis. Note displacement of epiphysis.

**Table 7.4**   Paediatric cervical spine injuries.

| Injury description | Radiographic diagnostic clues |
| --- | --- |
| Fracture through ring of C1 | • Loss of bony alignment<br>• Bilateral overhanging of lateral masses of C1 on C2 seen on antero-posterior projection<br>• Computed tomography (CT) may be useful |
| Torticollis (head tilting towards painful side) | • Spine tilted and rotated on antero-posterior projection<br>• Rotation of C1 on C2 on antero-posterior projection |
| Rotational subluxation at the atlanto-axial joint | • Rotational asymmetry of C1 lateral masses about odontoid peg on antero-posterior projection<br>• Condition usually self-limiting but if it fails to resolve, CT may be useful for assessment purposes |
| Odontoid peg fracture | • Results from acute hyperflexion (e.g. road traffic accident[23])<br>• Careful evaluation of odontoid peg on both lateral and antero-posterior projections necessary as injury may not disrupt the normal spinal alignments |
| C2/C3 fracture/subluxation | • Changes resemble pseudosubluxation but neck will not be held in flexion and other clinical symptoms will be apparent<br>• Associated vertebral fractures<br>• Disc space widening<br>• Prevertebral soft tissue swelling |

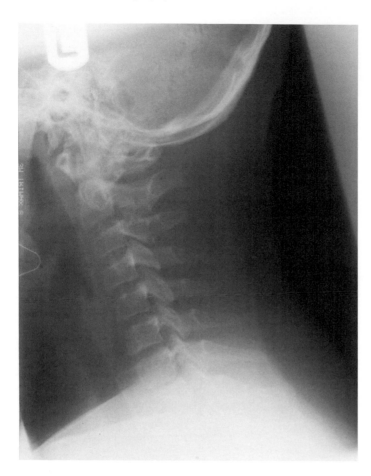

**Fig. 7.45**  Lateral cervical spine held in flexion. Note this positioning can create appearances of dislocation at the C2/C3/C4 level.

anterior to the odontoid peg which should be less than 5 mm in children, and an evaluation of the prevertebral soft tissues.

### The thoracolumbar spine

Skeletal injuries to the thoracolumbar spine result from high-powered forces and, in children under the age of 10 years, the mechanisms of trauma are typically a fall from a height, motor vehicle accidents or non-accidental injury. In older children and adolescents sporting injuries and accidents involving motor vehicles (e.g. motorcycles) tend to be the major associations[24].

'Wedge' fractures are the most common skeletal injury of the thoracolumbar spine. However, normal spinal development may result in apparent anterior wedging, particularly in the thoracic spine, and therefore the relative loss of vertebral height should be assessed in comparison to other neighbouring vertebrae. Severe axial compression can result in a 'burst' fracture of a lumbar vertebra with associated cord damage if backward movement (retropulsion) of the fracture fragments into the spinal canal occurs. 'Burst' fractures do not present in the thoracic spine as the thoracic curve prevents direct axial compression of the vertebrae.

Fractures of the lumbar transverse processes result generally from direct trauma and may be associated with internal abdominal injuries (e.g. kidney laceration). Identification of the psoas muscle shadow on the antero-posterior lumbar spine projection is important in these cases as obliteration of the psoas muscle shadow is suggestive of internal injury.

Plain film radiographic examination of the thoracolumbar spine should include an antero-posterior and a lateral projection. If further imaging is required then computed tomography (CT) is the imaging modality of choice to evaluate spinal trauma and this should be undertaken, even if plain film radiographs are negative, if clinical suspicion of skeletal trauma is high as occult or unusual injury patterns may have apparently normal plain film radiographic appearances.

## The pelvis

Pelvic fractures in children are uncommon. However, the mortality rate and the risk of medical complications are relatively high and therefore all pelvic

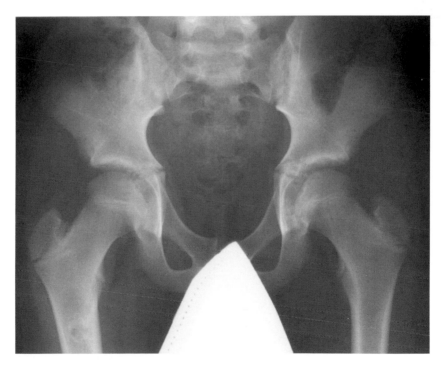

**Fig. 7.46** Pelvis radiograph following trauma. Asymmetry and apparent widening of the symphysis pubis. Note poor application of radiation protection obscures the area of interest.

radiographs for trauma need to be of a high technical standard to facilitate accurate clinical interpretation (Fig. 7.46).

The adult pelvis is essentially a rigid structure and pelvic compression will result in bony injury with possible associated internal soft tissue damage. The paediatric pelvis contains a greater amount of cartilage and is, therefore, more elastic than the adult pelvis and resilient to bony injury[6]. As a result, compression of the paediatric pelvis may not result in pelvic fractures but may still have associated internal soft tissue damage (e.g. haemorrhage, bladder or urethral damage). Specific pelvic injuries, including their radiographic appearances and associated injuries, are listed in Table 7.5.

Normal appearances and secondary ossification patterns of the paediatric pelvis can cause confusion and the radiographer should remember that the juvenile symphysis pubis and sacroiliac joints are frequently wider than those seen in adults. The triradiate cartilage of the acetabulum and the asymmetrically prominent ischiopubic ossification centres may also cause confusion due to their irregular appearances.

The radiographic projection of choice for initial evaluation of the pelvis is the antero-posterior projection with the femurs placed in internal rotation. Alternative imaging to investigate occult or complex injuries should be undertaken using CT.

**Table 7.5**  Pelvic injuries.

| Injury | Description/features |
|---|---|
| Ramus fracture | • May be single ramus or both rami, unilateral or bilateral<br>• Bilateral double ramus fracture = unstable ring fracture<br>• Unilateral double ramus fracture = stable pelvic ring break<br>• Associated injuries may be a disrupted symphysis or ruptured urethra or bladder |
| Apophyseal avulsion fracture | • Usually occurs at ischial tuberosity, anterior superior iliac spine (ASIS) or anterior inferior iliac spine (AIIS)<br>• Seen as a sports injury in adolescents (14 yrs +)<br>• AIIS avulsion may present as hip or groin pain |
| Iliac wing fracture | • Results from high-velocity trauma and is commonly seen in association with other skeletal injuries |
| Symphysis disruption | • Rare in children due to elasticity of paediatric pelvis<br>• May be seen as a component of multiple pelvic trauma |
| Anterior compression injuries | • Bilateral fractures of the pubic rami<br>• Opening and recoil of sacroiliac joints – not demonstrated radiographically |
| Lateral compression injuries | • Undisplaced fracture through the triradiate cartilage<br>• Pubic and ischial rami are laterally compressed +/– fracture<br>• Disruption of the ipsilateral sacroiliac joint |
| Vertical shear injuries | • Where one hemi pelvis rotates externally and is forced vertically<br>• Fractures of the pubic rami or diastasis of the symphysis accompanies subluxation of the sacroiliac joint<br>• Alternatively a vertical fracture may be seen lateral to the sacroiliac joint |

# Summary

Understanding paediatric trauma requires knowledge of paediatric growth patterns and developmental anatomy in order to be able to decipher the truly abnormal from a normal variation, and radiographers should have access to a textbook of normal developmental variants in their clinical working environment. This chapter has explored some of the common causes and appearances of paediatric skeletal trauma that may present themselves to radiographers working in the Accident and Emergency department. However, it is not exhaustive and radiographers are encouraged to discuss images with their radiological colleagues and read appropriate radiological texts and journals to improve their understanding of the subject. Uncommon or subtle skeletal injuries can easily be missed but the application of the simple radiographic evaluation tools introduced in this chapter will assist the radiographer in their clinical practice and improve their confidence and ability to recognise paediatric skeletal trauma.

# References

1. Hardy, M. (2000) Paediatric radiography: is there a need for postgraduate education? *Radiography* **6**, 27–34.
2. Rogers, L.F. (1992) *Radiology of Skeletal Trauma,* 2nd edn. Churchill Livingstone, New York.
3. Raby, N., Berman, L. and de lacey, G. (1995) *Accident & Emergency Radiology, A Survival Guide.* WB Saunders Company, London.
4. Donnelly, L.F., Klostermeier, T.T. and Klostermeier, L.A. (1998) Traumatic elbow effusions in paediatrics: are occult fractures the rule? *American Journal of Roengenology* **171** (1), 243–5.
5. Manaster, B.J. (1997) *Handbook of Skeletal Radiology,* 2nd edn. Mosby, London.
6. Carty, H., Shaw, D., Brunelle, F. and Kendall, B. (eds) (1994) *Imaging Children*, Volume 2. Churchill Livingstone, London.
7. Thornton, A. and Gyll, C. (1999) *Children's fractures.* WB Saunders Company, Harcourt Publishers, London.
8. Angermann, P. and Lohmann, M. (1993) Injuries to the hand and wrist – a study of 50,272 injuries. *Journal of Hand Surgery – British Volume* **18** (5), 642–4.
9. Hove, L.M. (1993) Fractures of the hand. Distribution and relative incidence. *Scandinavian Journal of Plastic and Reconstructive Surgery and Hand Surgery* **27** (4), 317–19.
10. Rajesh, A., Basu, A., Vaidhyanath, R. and Finlay, D. (2001) Hand fractures: a study of their site and type in childhood. *Clinical Radiology* **56**, 667–9.
11. Bhende, M.S., Dandrea, L.A. and Davis, L.W. (1993) Hand injuries in children presenting to a pediatric emergency department. *Annals of Emergency Medicine* **2** (10), 1519–23.
12. De Jonge, J.J., Kingma, J., van der Lei, B. *et al.* (1994) Phalangeal fractures of the hand. An analysis of gender and age related incidence and aetiology. *Journal of Hand Surgery – British Volume* **19** (2), 168–70.
13. Buhari, S.A., Singh, S., Wong, H.P. *et al.* (1993) Tibial tuberosity fractures in adolescents. *Singapore Medical Journal* **34** (5), 421–4.

14. John, S.D., Moorthy, C.S and Swischuk, L.E. (1997) Expanding the concept of the toddler's fracture. *Radiographics* **17** (2), 367–76.
15. Koury, S.I., Stone, C.K., Harrell, G. *et al.* (1999) Recognition and management of Tillaux fractures in adolescents. *Paediatric Emergency Care* **15** (1), 37–9.
16. Steinlauf, S.D., Stricker, S.J. and Hulen, C.A. (1998) Juvenile Tillaux fracture simulating syndesmosis separation: a case report. *Foot and Ankle International* **19** (5), 332–5.
17. Chande, V.T. (1995) Decision rules for roentgenography of children with acutre ankle injuries. *Archives of Paediatrics and Adolescent Medicine* **149** (3), 225–8.
18. Blumberg, K. and Patterson, R.J. (1991) The toddler's cuboid fracture. *Radiology* **179** (1), 93–4.
19. Owen, R.J., Hickey, F.G. and Finlay, D.B. (1995) A study of metatarsal fractures in children. *Injury* **26** (8), 537–8.
20. Schwartz, G.R., Wright, S.W., Fein, J.A. *et al.* (1997) Paediatric cervical spine injury sustained in falls from low heights. *Annals of Emergency Medicine* **30** (3), 249–52.
21. Rooks, V.J., Sisler, C. and Burton, B. (1998) Cervical spine injury in child abuse: report of two cases. *Paediatric Radiology* **28** (3), 193–5.
22. Kleiman, P.K. and Shelton, Y.A. (1997) Hangman's fracture in an abused infant: imaging features. *Paediatric Radiology* **27** (9), 776–7.
23. Blauth, M., Schmidt, U., Otte, D. *et al.* (1996) Fractures of the odontoid process in small children: biomechanical analysis and report of three cases. *European Spine Journal* **5** (1), 63–70.
24. Phaltankar, P.M. and Patel, B.R. (1997) Fracture-dislocation at the thoraco-lumbar junction in an infant with locked vertebrae. A case report. *Spine* **22** (16), 1933–5.

# Chapter 8
# Orthopaedics

Congenital and developmental skeletal abnormalities may occur as a result of many embryonic, chromosomal, developmental, hereditary and metabolic disorders. However, the exact cause (aetiology) of many of these conditions is unknown. The role of imaging is often fundamental in the diagnosis, treatment and management of patients with skeletal abnormalities and all imaging modalities may have a valuable role to play (Table 8.1).

**Table 8.1**　Role of imaging in paediatric orthopaedics.

| Imaging modality | Advantages | Disadvantages |
| --- | --- | --- |
| Plain film radiography | • Initial imaging investigation<br>• Provides a gross anatomy baseline<br>• Relatively inexpensive | • Cannot detect subtle reductions in bone density. 30–50% bone loss required before osteopenic changes can be seen |
| Computed tomography (CT) | • Demonstrates bone and soft tissue<br>• Computed image manipulation can enhance bony and soft tissue lesions<br>• Contrast agents can enhance lesions | • Need to sedate or anaesthetise a young child<br>• Relatively high dose and cost |
| Magnetic resonance imaging (MRI) | • Excellent soft tissue detail<br>• No exposure to ionising radiation | • Bone detail relatively poor<br>• Need to sedate or anaesthetise a young child<br>• Relatively expensive |
| Ultrasound | • High sensitivity in the detection of effusions in superficial joints<br>• Dynamic evaluation of joints possible<br>• Good soft tissue differentiation, will demonstrate non-ossified cartilaginous epiphyses without need for contrast agents[1]<br>• No exposure to ionising radiation or need for sedation<br>• Relatively inexpensive | • Technique, quality of examination and interpretation are operator dependent<br>• Visualisation of deep-seated structures may be limited |
| Scintigraphy | • Has a broad scope of clinical applications<br>• Useful for identifying multifocal lesions<br>• More sensitive than plain film radiography as detects changes in bone metabolism resulting in early identification of pathology | • Non-specific investigation – findings need to be correlated with results of other imaging modalities<br>• Low to moderate radiation dose in comparison to plain film radiography. However, benefit of increased sensitivity outweighs associated risks |

This chapter will consider a range of common or diagnostically important paediatric orthopaedic conditions, including skeletal infections and neoplasms, and examine the use and value of diagnostic imaging in the assessment of these conditions.

# The foot

The accurate imaging of paediatric foot disorders is essential in order to direct appropriate treatment. Many clinicians will require the foot to be imaged while weight bearing, and in non-ambulant infants this will require the child to be positioned supine or seated with the knee(s) held in flexion (Fig. 8.1). The guardian should then hold the proximal tibia and place downward pressure on the foot to simulate weight bearing[2]. Additional CT or MRI examinations may also be required in young children to evaluate the non-ossified cartilaginous tarsus[3].

## *Metatarsus adductus/varus*

Metatarsus adductus is a common foot deformity that is characterised by incurving of the forefoot. The condition is bilateral in up to 50% of patients[4] and, as the foot retains its flexibility, the majority of cases resolve spontaneously without medical intervention. In contrast, metatarsus varus is an uncommon condition (10% of cases) that results in outcurving of the forefoot. This condition is often rigid and persists into adulthood.

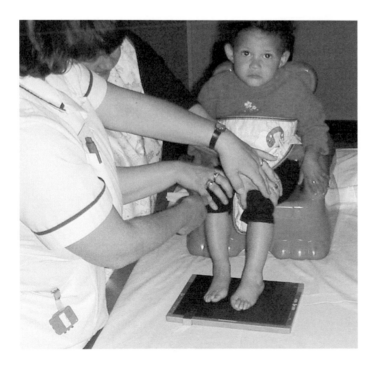

**Fig. 8.1** Child positioned for simulated weight-bearing dorsi-plantar foot. Note the radiographer clearly demonstrating the required positioning to the guardian.

### *Talipes equinovarus (club foot)*

Talipes equinovarus is a relatively common congenital foot abnormality and is found in approximately 1 in 1000 live births[4,5]. The condition presents bilaterally in 50% of cases and is believed to result from a combination of intrauterine and genetic factors, although exact aetiology is unknown. Radiographic examination should include a dorsi-plantar projection with simulated weight bearing and a horizontal beam lateral projection[6]. Assessment of the dorsi-plantar radiograph will demonstrate a decreased talocalcaneal angle as a result of the navicular and cuboid being medially displaced relative to the talus and calcaneum (Figs 8.2–8.4). Delayed ossification of the talus and calcaneum may also be seen[7]. On the lateral projection the metatarsals appear to lie above one another with the talus and calcaneum approximately parallel.

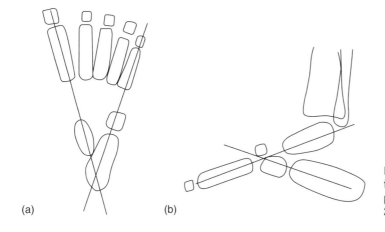

(a)  (b)

**Fig. 8.2** (a) and (b) Normal talocalcaneal angle on the dorsi-plantar foot should be between 20° and 40°.

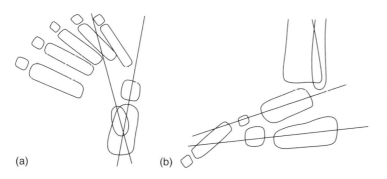

(a)  (b)

**Fig. 8.3** (a) and (b) Talipes equinovarus. Note the talocalcaneal angle is markedly reduced (<20°) on dorsi-plantar projection and the parallel orientation of the talus and calcaneum on the lateral projection.

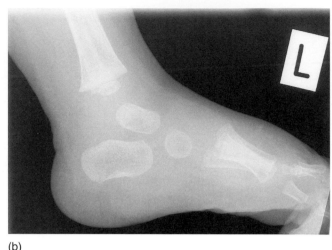

(b)

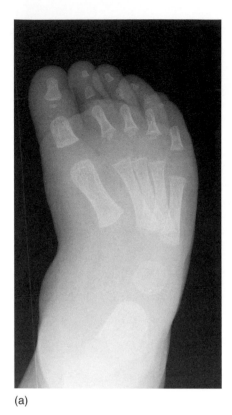

(a)

**Fig. 8.4**   (a) and (b) Talipes equinovarus.

### Pes planus (flat foot)

Physiological flat feet are present in nearly all infants, many children and approximately 15% of adults[5]. It is thought to be a hereditary condition associated with a valgus heel and decreased height of the longitudinal arch. Imaging is not required unless the condition becomes painful and requires orthopaedic intervention.

### Osteochondrosis and osteochondritis

Osteochondrosis is the idiopathic avascular necrosis and regeneration of epiphyses that occurs with growth[5] whereas osteochondritis is the inflammation of both bone and cartilage that occurs secondary to the disruption of the vascular supply to the bone, probably as a result of repetitive trauma. Clinically and radiographically, the two conditions are indistinguishable with patients presenting with localised pain and tenderness while radiographs demonstrate varying stages of fragmentation and regeneration (Figs 8.5–8.7). As a result, many texts use the terms synonymously to describe apparent spontaneous avascular necrosis in childhood and adolescence.

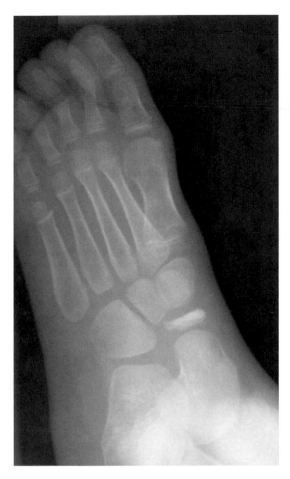

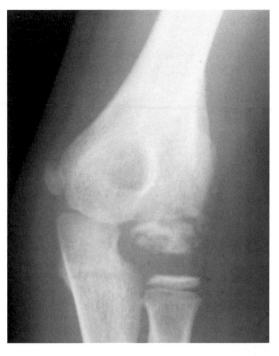

**Fig. 8.6**   Panner's disease – osteochondritis of the capitellum.

**Fig. 8.5**   Köhler's disease – osteochondritis of the navicular bone. Note the compressed shape and marked increased density.

# The knee and lower leg

## Osgood-Schlatter disease

Osgood-Schlatter disease is essentially traction apophysitis of the tibial tubercle that occurs in adolescent children as a result of repetitive micro trauma and overuse[5]. Clinical presentation is typically prolonged intermittent pain over the tibial tubercle with symptoms generally subsiding following fusion of the apophyseal growth plate[4]. Occasionally the tubercle will remain unfused and

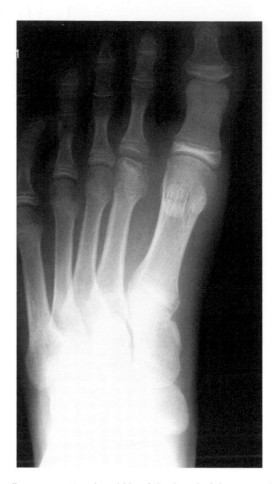

**Fig. 8.7**   Freiberg's disease – osteochondritis of the head of the second metatarsal.

fragmented[7], but as the condition is normally self-limiting, imaging is not routinely required.

### Sinding-Larson-Johansson syndrome

This syndrome is commonly thought to be traction apophysitis of the distal pole of the patella and has been fondly termed 'jumper's knee'. The distal pole of the patella is typically cartilaginous, and distraction and fragmented ossification can occur following tensile loading through the quadriceps mechanism. A joint effusion may also be noted with this condition[4].

### Tibial bowing

Tibial bowing is a common and varied abnormality, the morbidity of the condition being dependent upon the direction of the tibial apex (the point of the bow).

Lateral bowing is seen commonly in infants and is thought to be a variation of normal. Appearances are typically bilateral and symmetrical and diagnostic imaging examinations are not routinely required. Anterior and postero-medial bowing are both uncommon conditions that result in limb shortening. Anterior bowing is also associated with fibula hemimelia whereas postero-medial bowing may have associated foot abnormalities. Antero-lateral bowing has serious prognostic implications, as a spontaneous increase in tibial bowing will result in a fracture at the tibial apex and possible pseudarthrosis[5] (Fig. 8.8).

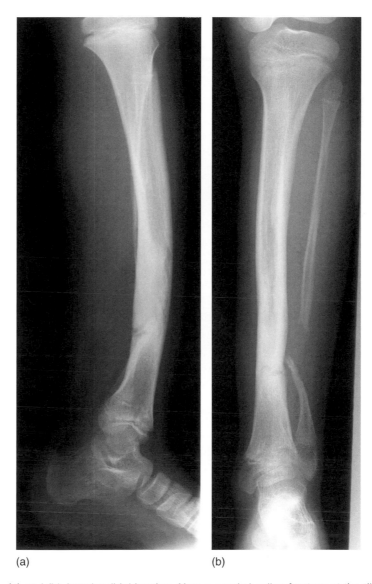

(a)                              (b)

**Fig. 8.8**   (a) and (b) Anterior tibial bowing. Note a poorly healing fracture at the tibial apex is associated with pseudarthrosis of the fibula.

**Box 8.1**   Paediatric hip: the role of imaging.

> *Plain film radiography*
> - First choice for assessment of slipped capital femoral epiphysis
> - Useful to assess the severity of Perthes' disease
>
> *Ultrasound*
> - Useful to identify and assess developmental dysplasia of the hip
>
> *Scintigraphy*
> - May identify a radiographically occult source of pain/disease/trauma
>
> *Magnetic resonance imaging (MRI)*
> - Useful in the early detection of avascular necrosis
> - Permits early diagnosis of tumours about the pelvis
>
> *Computed tomography (CT)*
> - Accurate evaluation of acetabular fractures

# The hip

Hip problems in children are relatively common and early diagnosis is important to prevent long-term morbidity and disability[8]. All imaging modalities may have a role to play in the diagnosis of paediatric hip conditions (Box 8.1).

## Transient synovitis

Transient synovitis, also known as toxic synovitis or irritable hip, is an acute inflammatory arthritis of unknown aetiology. Usually presenting unilaterally, it is the commonest cause of an acute limp and pain in children under 10 years of age[9]. Ultrasound is the imaging modality of choice in the diagnosis of transient synovitis and the condition normally resolves over a period of 2 weeks if the joint is allowed to rest. Follow-up plain film radiography is necessary if the symptoms return or fail to resolve as recurrent transient synovitis is associated with Perthes' disease (2–3% of cases)[5,9,10].

## Developmental dysplasia of the hip

Developmental dysplasia of the hip (DDH) is a generic term used to describe a spectrum of anatomical hip abnormalities[5]. The exact aetiology of hip dysplasia is unknown but thought to be multifactorial in nature with the majority of cases probably related to ligamentous laxity *in utero* induced by maternal hormones, although a breech intrauterine presentation and positive family history are also recognised risk factors[2,4,5]. Early diagnosis of hip dysplasia is critical if long-term disability is to be avoided and, therefore, it is routine practice in the UK for a physical examination of the neonate's hips to be undertaken by a paediatric physician within a few days of birth. Where the physical examination is positive, ultrasound assessment should be undertaken[11] to assess the anatomical position of the cartilaginous femoral head relative to the acetabulum[1].

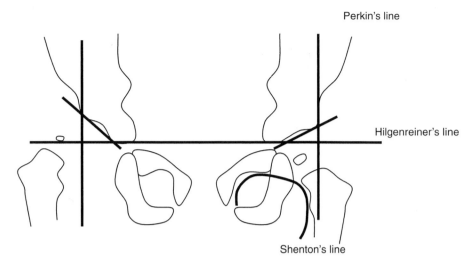

Perkin's line

Hilgenreiner's line

Shenton's line

**Fig. 8.9** Assessment of developmental dysplasia of the hip on a plain film radiograph of the pelvis. The femoral head should be seen within the lower medial quadrant of the cross made by Hilgenreiner's line and Perkin's line.

Ultrasound is the imaging modality of choice to assess the hip of a neonate or young infant but its role in the management of hip dysplasia declines with the increasing ossification of the femoral head as this reflects the beam and prevents accurate assessment of the acetabulum. In older infants, plain film radiography of the hip and pelvis are therefore requested in preference to ultrasound. The Von Rosen projection, which is still described in many radiological texts, is no longer recommended[6]. Instead, radiographic diagnosis of DDH is undertaken on an antero-posterior projection of the pelvis with the feet positioned vertically and follows careful evaluation of the position of the ossified femoral epiphysis relative to Hilgenreiner's line (a horizontal line connecting the supero-lateral borders of the triradiate cartilages), Perkin's line (a vertical line through the lateral rim of the acetabulum) and Shenton's line (an arc formed by the medial surface of the proximal femur and the inferior margin of the superior pubic ramus) and the acetabular angle which, if greater than 30°, is highly suggestive of dysplasia[12] (Figs 8.9 and 8.10).

## Perthes' disease

Legg-Calvé-Perthes' disease is the idiopathic juvenile avascular necrosis of the femoral head[5]. It presents more frequently in boys than girls (M:F = 4:1) and is normally unilateral, although non-simultaneous bilateral presentations have been noted in 10–20% of cases[4,5]. The mean age of onset is 7 years. Although the exact cause of the disease onset is unknown, the necrotic changes result from an interruption in the blood supply causing reduced femoral head ossification, fragmentation and ultimate deformation. A child with Perthes' disease will commonly present with an acute limp and scintigraphy, MRI and plain film radiography may all have a role to play in the initial assessment[5,13] (Fig. 8.11).

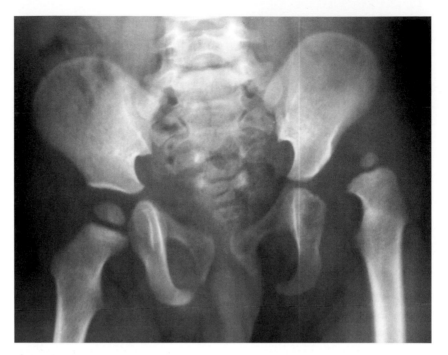

**Fig. 8.10**   Developmental dysplasia of the hip. Obvious displacement of the femoral head outside of the acetabulum. Note delayed ossification of the affected femoral head.

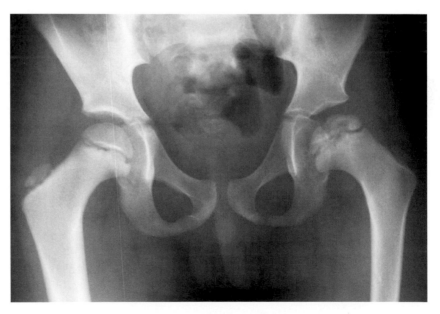

**Fig. 8.11**   Perthes' disease. Note fragmentation of the femoral epiphysis and apparent widening of the joint space.

### Slipped capital femoral epiphysis

The slipped capital femoral epiphysis (SCFE) is typically gradual in onset although it may occasionally occur acutely following a fall. It is predominantly seen in males (M:F = 3:1) between the ages of 9 and 15 years, and has been linked with the period of rapid growth during puberty and the associated weakening of the epiphyseal plate as a result of increased growth hormone levels. Individuals prone to SCFE tend to be obese, with up to 50% having evidence of endocrine disturbance. A radiographic diagnosis of SCFE on an antero-posterior pelvis radiograph is possible if widening of the physeal plate and postero-medial movement of the epiphysis relative to the femoral metaphysis can be identified (Fig. 8.12). Unfortunately, unless severe, an SCFE may not always be obvious on the antero-posterior pelvis projection and although Klein's lines may be a useful diagnostic tool (Fig. 8.13), a lateral projection of the hip is required to confirm diagnosis (Fig. 8.14).

## The upper limb

### Sprengel's deformity

Sprengel's deformity is the congenital elevation of the scapula as a result of the shoulder girdle failing to descend from its embryonic position in the neck[7] (Fig. 8.15). It is normally unilateral in presentation and may be associated with other orthopaedic conditions (e.g. Klippel-Feil syndrome, cervical spina bifida).

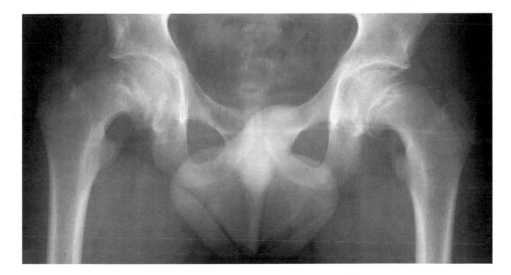

**Fig. 8.12** Bilateral slipped capital femoral epiphysis.

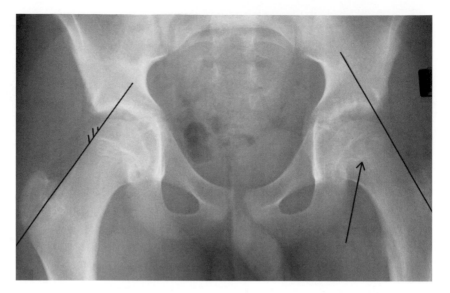

**Fig. 8.13**   Klein's lines drawn along the lateral border of the femoral neck should intersect with the outer portion of the femoral epiphyses. Failure to do so is suggestive of slipped capital femoral epiphysis and a lateral projection should be undertaken to confirm diagnosis.

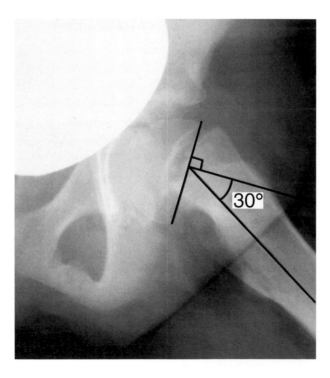

**Fig. 8.14**   Lateral projection of the hip clearly shows the postero-medial displacement of the femoral epiphysis.

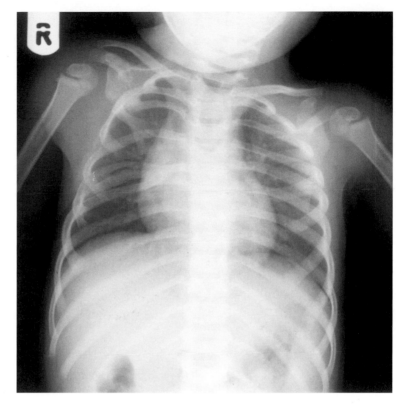

**Fig. 8.15** Sprengel's deformity. Note the high lying position of the scapula.

## The radius and ulna

Radial and ulnar defects are varied in presentation and severity, with radial abnormalities being more common than those of the ulna (Fig. 8.16). Deformities include radioulnar synostosis, where fusion between the proximal radius and ulna occurs, radial or ulna club hand, as a result of absence or hypoplasia of the radius/ulna and associated musculature, and madelung deformity, where shortening and bowing of the radius results in posterior dislocation of the normally shaped ulna at the wrist and abnormal radial articulation with the carpus.

## Polydactyly and syndactyly

Polydactyly (duplication of fingers or toes) is a common abnormality and is usually inherited as an autosomal dominant characteristic (Fig. 8.17). Syndactyly is the fusion of the fingers or toes (Fig. 8.18). Both polydactyly and syndactyly can involve bone or soft tissue and both may require surgery in later childhood for cosmetic purposes.

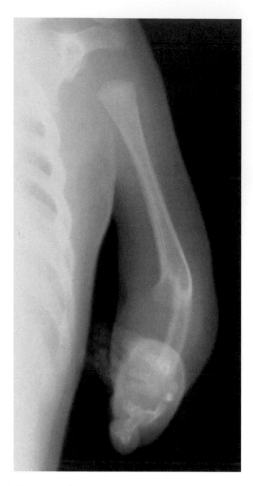

**Fig. 8.16**   Humero-radial synostosis.

# The spine

Back pain in children is uncommon[5] and because of the potential for spinal disease to result in considerable disability, accurate assessment and diagnosis of all spinal complaints is essential and MRI, in the majority of cases, is the imaging modality of choice[14].

## Discitis

Discitis is an infrequent problem of the paediatric thoracolumbar spine[15] that results from bacterial infection of the intervertebral disc spreading to the vertebral endplates of the adjacent vertebrae over a period of several weeks[12]. Clinical symptoms are dependent upon patient age and include fever and vomiting in the younger child, while in adolescents back pain is the most common presentation. Plain film radiography of the spine will demonstrate a reduced

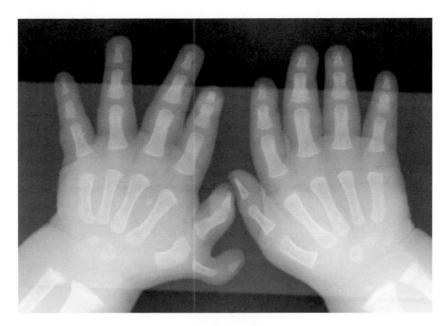

**Fig. 8.17** Polydactyly – shown here is duplication of the thumb of the left hand.

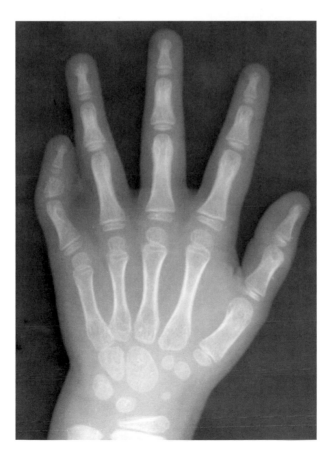

**Fig. 8.18** Syndactyly – shown here is soft tissue webbing of the fourth and fifth fingers.

intervertebral disc height approximately 2–4 weeks post onset of the infection. However, in all cases MRI is the imaging modality of choice (Fig. 8.19).

## Kyphosis and lordosis

Paediatric kyphosis and lordosis are uncommon when compared to scoliosis. A possible cause of increased kyphosis and reduced lumbar lordosis during early adolescence is Scheuermann's disease which results in the anterior compression of the vertebral body. Plain film radiographic examination should include an antero-posterior and a lateral projection. However, it is essential that the arms are not raised above the level of the lower costal margin as this will considerably alter the normal spinal curvature and invalidate the diagnostic accuracy of the examination[16].

## Scoliosis

Scoliosis is defined as the lateral curvature of the spine although a sagittal or transverse component to the curve may also be present. The majority of childhood scoliosis cases are idiopathic in nature[17] (i.e. of unknown cause) with the age of scoliosis onset being directly related to the severity of the curve at skeletal maturity[7] (Fig. 8.20). Despite technological advancements, plain film radiography is still the examination of choice to provide the initial diagnosis and evaluate the degree of the curve. However, MRI also has a significant role to play, particularly in the assessment of intraspinal anomalies and pre-surgical planning[18].

Plain film radiographic examination of the spine for scoliosis should be performed with the patient erect, and a single antero-posterior or postero-anterior projection of the whole spine is sufficient for diagnosis and observational monitoring of curves less than 20°[16]. However, as patients with progressive scoliosis may have regular imaging to assess the progression of the curve, it is important that the radiation dose is minimised and to facilitate this, the postero-anterior projection is preferred as it will reduce the dose to the sensitive anterior organs. The adoption of a high kilovoltage technique will also reduce patient dose whilst facilitating the visualisation of the whole spine.

The lower border of the cassette should be positioned at the level of the anterior superior iliac spines and collimation opened to include the whole of the spine and the iliac crests. Skeletal maturity is achieved when the iliac crest apophyses reach the posterior superior iliac spines and therefore these should be included on all assessment radiographs[7]. Where radiographs of non-ambulatory patients are requested then these should be undertaken with the spine in its normal functional position (i.e. sitting or supine). In cases where the patient presents symptomatically (e.g. back pain) then additional lateral or oblique projections may be required; however, these should not be undertaken routinely.

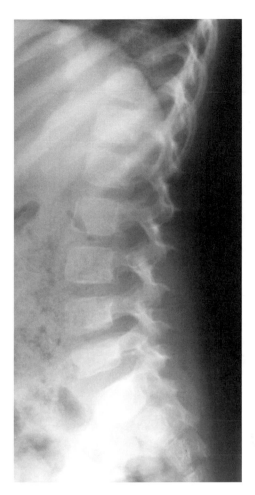

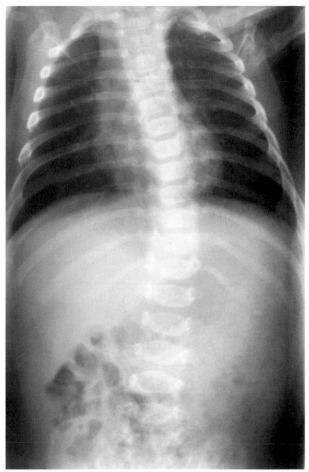

**Fig. 8.19** Juvenile discitis. Note narrowing of the L4/L5 joint space.

**Fig. 8.20** Idiopathic scoliosis.

# Infection

Infection of the musculoskeletal system can cause severe disability if not detected and treated at an early stage and all imaging modalities may have a role to play (Box 8.2).

The clinical history provided by the patient or their family can provide important clues to infection, and signs of systemic illness, localised swelling, erythema, reduction in limb movement or unusual limb position are all suggestive of an infective process.

## Osteomyelitis

Osteomyelitis commonly occurs as a result of haematogenous spread (via the blood) and may be acute, subacute or chronic in presentation. It is typically seen

**Box 8.2**    The role of imaging in the detection and treatment of musculoskeletal infection[19].

---

*Plain film radiography*
- Preliminary examination to exclude trauma or other pathologies

*Ultrasound*
- Useful in the detection of joint effusions and fluid collections in the soft tissues and sub-periosteal regions
- May guide aspiration or drainage of fluid collections or effusions

*Scintigraphy*
- Has a high sensitivity rate and is useful in the identification of multifocal infection

*Magnetic resonance imaging (MRI)*
- High sensitivity
- Can accurately assess soft tissues and bones to evaluate the local extent of musculoskeletal infections

*Computed tomography (CT)*
- Can detect osseous or soft tissue abnormalities, particularly gas in the soft tissues

---

in the metaphyseal region of long bones as a result of the slow movement of blood through the sinusoidal vessels which allows bacteria to adhere to the vascular membranes. Clinical symptoms of osteomyelitis include localised pain and swelling and a recent history of systemic illness (e.g. ear or chest infection). Radiographic findings depend upon the age of the patient and the time of infection onset. However, plain films are not sensitive to early osteomyelitic changes and although they may be requested to exclude other causes of the patient's symptoms, scintigraphy is the initial imaging investigation of choice in cases of suspected skeletal infection[7] (Fig. 8.21).

### Septic arthritis

Septic arthritis is the inflammation of a joint as a result of infection. The infection may enter the joint directly (traumatic or surgical infection), or indirectly from an adjacent osteomyelitic infection or by haematogenous spread. Clinical symptoms include local or systemic illness and localised swelling and tenderness. The child may also resist movement of the affected limb and maintain it in a flexed position. Ultrasound may be used to identify synovial thickening and joint effusion in the early stages of septic arthritis. However, MRI is the imaging modality of choice.

## Bone tumours

The majority of paediatric bone tumours are benign in nature and most have specific and characteristic radiographic or clinical presentations, therefore permitting accurate diagnosis without the need of a biopsy[20]. Malignant bone tumours

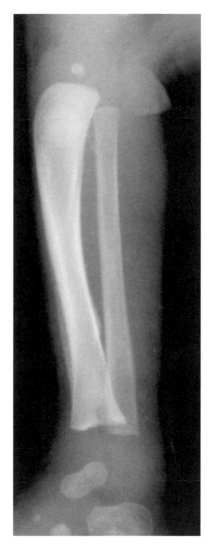

**Fig. 8.21**   Osteomyelitic changes in the left distal tibia. Note distal tibial lucency and raised periosteum.

are relatively rare when compared to other paediatric malignancies, and the large majority are osteosarcoma (60%)[21] and Ewing's sarcoma (30%)[22] although it should be noted that up to 20% of children with leukaemia present with bone pain[5].

## Fibrous cortical defect and non-ossifying fibroma

Fibrous cortical defects are fibrous lesions of the bone, commonly noted as incidental findings, and are usually accepted as a variation of normal. They are typically small, well-delineated, asymptomatic lesions found within the cortex of the

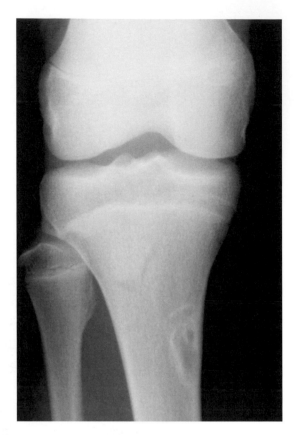

**Fig. 8.22**   Non-ossifying fibroma in proximal tibia.

bone and tend to resolve spontaneously. The non-ossifying fibroma is a larger version of the fibrous cortical defect (Fig. 8.22).

### Fibrous dysplasia

Fibrous dysplasia occurs as a result of medullary bone being replaced by well-defined areas of fibrous tissue and fluid-filled cysts[7]. The cause of fibrous dysplasia is unknown and lesions are often asymptomatic and noted as an incidental finding unless a pathological fracture through the lesion has occurred. Commonly affected bones are the pelvis, femur, ribs and skull. Plain film radiographic appearances include bone expansion and scalloping of the cortical margins (Fig. 8.23).

### Osteochondroma

The osteochondroma is essentially an osseous growth arising from the bony metaphyseal cortex[7] and is usually first noted as a painful mass following a direct blow[5]. It occurs commonly around the knee and proximal humerus, and is accurately diagnosed using plain film radiography (Fig. 8.24).

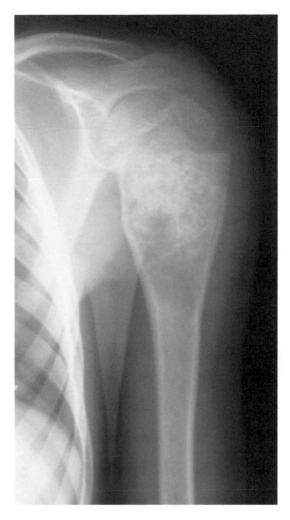

**Fig. 8.23** Fibrous dysplasia in proximal humerus.

## Enchondroma

Enchondromas are commonly found in the phalanges and long bones, and cause bone expansion and cortical thinning. A pathological fracture through the lesion may occur as a result of bone weakness.

## Chondroblastoma

A chondroblastoma is a rare tumour found in the epiphysis and may produce an inflammatory reaction suggestive of infective arthritis. Clinical presentation is typically mild joint pain with limited movement. Plain film radiographs will demonstrate a well-defined radiolucent lesion within the epiphysis.

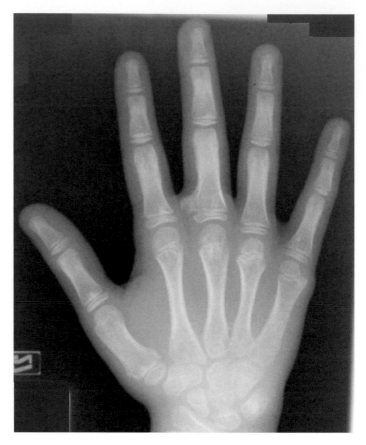

**Fig. 8.24**   Metaphyseal bony outgrowths.

### Osteoid osteoma

Osteoid osteomas are bone-forming tumours that are typically described on radiographs as having a central radiolucent nidus surrounded by a reactive sclerosis. The charcteristic clinical symptoms of night pain relieved by aspirin support the radiographic diagnosis and further imaging is not generally required.

### Solitary/unicameral bone cyst

The solitary bone cyst is a common benign bone lesion that presents initially within the metaphyseal region and migrates towards the diaphysis with bone growth. It is generally asymptomatic in nature and usually only presents following a pathological fracture through the lesion. Radiographically, it is defined as an expansile lesion with well-defined margins that may be multilocular in appearance. Treatment is by steroid injection and the previously recommended treatment of curettage and bone grafting is now rarely required (Fig. 8.25).

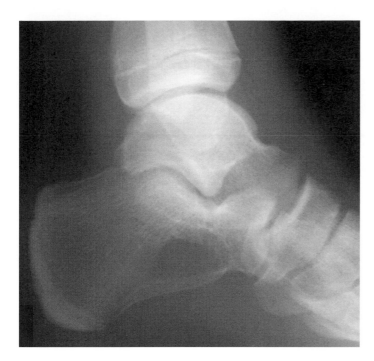

**Fig. 8.25** Calcaneal cyst.

## Osteosarcoma

The osteosarcoma is the most common primary malignant bone tumour of childhood and commonly presents during the adolescent period as localised pain and swelling. Fifty per cent of lesions occur around the knee and plain film radiographs will demonstrate altered bone density and a 'frayed' periosteal reaction (Fig. 8.26). Scintigraphy is the imaging modality of choice to assess metastatic spread whereas MRI will evaluate the extent of local bone and soft tissue involvement. Treatment is by resection and aggressive chemotherapy.

## Ewing's sarcoma

Ewing's sarcoma is a rapidly progressive malignant bone lesion that presents with localised pain and swelling but also signs of systemic illness. The lesions are often found in the long bones of children, although they may also be located in the axial skeleton of adolescents and older children. Metastatic spread is generally to the lungs and other bones and the aggressive nature of the lesion results in a relatively poor prognosis with only 50–60% of patients surviving 5 years despite resection of the tumour and aggressive chemotherapy. Plain film radiographic appearances of the lesion are often non-specific and CT/MRI and scintigraphy are the imaging examinations of choice to assess the local extent of the lesion and metastatic spread.

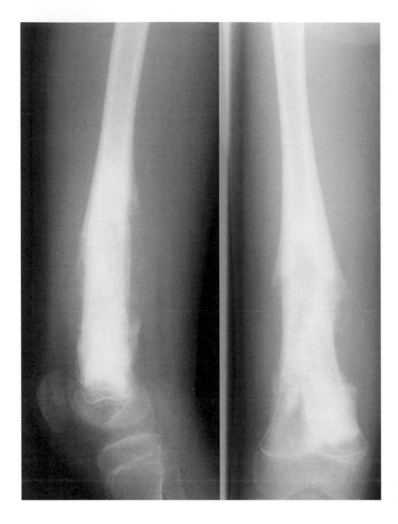

**Fig. 8.26**  Osteosarcoma of the distal femur.

## Summary

Radiographic examination of children with skeletal abnormalities is often essential in deciding appropriate patient management and treatment. This chapter has introduced a number of common or diagnostically important paediatric orthopaedic conditions and has described their likely radiographic appearances and, where appropriate, provided guidelines on imaging protocols, including the value of alternative imaging modalities in the diagnosis of skeletal pathology.

## References

1. Sanders, R.C. (1998) *Clinical Sonography: A Practical Guide*, 3rd edn. Lippincott-Raven, New York.
2. Carty, H., Shaw, D., Brunelle, F. and Kendall, B. (eds) (1994) *Imaging Children*. Churchill Livingstone, London.

3.  Harty, M.P. (2001) Imaging of pediatric foot disorders. *Radiologic Clinics of North America* **39** (4), 738–48.

4.  Chew, F.S. (1997) *Skeletal Radiology: The Bare Bones*, 2nd edn. Williams & Wilkins, London.

5.  Staheli, L.T. (1998) *Fundamentals of Pediatric Orthopaedics.* Lippincott-Raven, New York.

6.  Gyll, C. and Blake, N. (1986) *Paediatric Diagnostic Imaging.* William Heinemann Medical Books, London.

7.  Sutton, D. (ed.) (1998) *Textbook of Radiology and Imaging*, 6th edn. Churchill Livingstone, London.

8.  Hubbard, A.M. and Dormans, J.P. (1995) Evaluation of developmental dysplasia, Perthes' disease, and neuromuscular dysplasia of the hip in children before and after surgery: an imaging update. *American Journal of Roentgenology* **164** (5), 1067–73.

9.  Waters, E. (1995) Toxic synovitis of the hip in children. *Nurse Practitioner* **20** (4), 44–51.

10. Wingstrand, H. (1999) Significance of synovitis in Legg-Calvé-Perthes disease. *Journal of Pediatric Orthopaedics. Part B* **8** (3), 156–60.

11. Apley, A.G. and Solomon, L. (1994) *Concise System of Orthopaedics and Fractures*, 2nd edn. Butterworth-Heinnemann, Oxford.

12. Dähnert, W. (2000) *Radiology Review Manual*, 4th edn. Lippincott Williams & Wilkins, London.

13. Connolly, L.P. and Treves, S.T. (1998) Assessing the limping child with skeletal scintigraphy. *Journal of Nuclear Medicine* **39** (6), 1056–61.

14. Egelhoff, J.C. (1999) MR imaging of congenital anomalies of the paediatric spine. *Magnetic Resonance Imaging Clinics of North America* **7** (3), 459–79.

15. Fernandez, M., Carrol, C.L. and Baker, C.J. (2000) Discitis and vertebral osteomyelitis in children: an 18 year review. *Pediatrics* **105** (6), 1299–304.

16. Weinstein, S. (2001) *The Pediatric Spine: Principles and Practice*, 2nd edn. Lippincott Williams & Wilkins, London.

17. Kim, F.M., Poussaint, T.Y. and Barnes, P.D. (1999) Neuroimaging of scoliosis in childhood. *Neuroimaging Clinics of North America* **9** (1), 195–221.

18. Redla, S., Sikdar, T. and Saifuddin, A. (2001) Magnetic resonance imaging of scoliosis. *Clinical Radiology* **56,** 360–71.

19. Kothari, N.A., Pelchovitz, D.J. and Meyer, J.S. (2001) Imaging of musculoskeletal infections. *Radiologic Clinics of North America* **39** (4), 653–71.

20. Aboulafia, A.J., Kennon, R.E. and Jelinek, J.S. (1999) Benign bone tumors of childhood. *Journal of the American Academy of Orthopaedic Surgeons* **7** (6), 377–88.

21. Davies, A.M. (2001) Imaging in skeletal oncology. *European Journal of Radiology* **37**, 79–94.

22. St Jude Children's Research Hospital. *Ewing Sarcoma.* http://www.StJude.org/medical/ewing.htm

# Chapter 9
# Non-accidental injury

Child abuse is a persistent societal problem that has transcended the centuries[1]. It is currently separated into four different categories: physical, sexual and emotional abuse, and neglect (see Box 9.1) but each is not mutually exclusive and it has been argued that emotional abuse is inherent in all of the other abuse categories[3]. Clinical suspicion of physical abuse (non-accidental injury) will generally result in the patient being referred for radiographic imaging to assist in diagnosis and it is this category of abuse that this chapter aims to expand upon. However, an appreciation of the other abuse classifications (and how to recognise them) would be advantageous to any health care professional working with children.

How physical abuse is differentiated from an acceptable degree of parental control is not internationally consistent. It is influenced by environmental and cultural traditions and, in a multicultural society, these may cause conflict between the social services and cultural leaders. However, it is generally accepted that abuse is determined from a societal perspective and therefore parental discipline becomes abuse when the expectations and rules of society are contravened[4].

Over recent years, the reported incidences of physical child abuse have increased[5] and yet the number of children placed upon the child protection register as a result of physical abuse has decreased[6]. This is likely to be due to a change in government social policy from the sanctioning and stigmatisation of children and their families by removing children into care, to working together with families to improve parenting skills.

## Physical abuse

Physical abuse victims are commonly young children with 80% of reported incidences involving children under the age of 2 years[7]. The sex of the child does not appear to affect the likelihood of physical abuse but other risk factors have been identified and these are summarised in Box 9.2.

## Role of imaging

Non-accidental injury (NAI) frequently presents via the Accident and Emergency department as either an occult injury or as a raised clinical suspicion due to unclear and inappropriate history or other suspicious signs[7] (see Box 9.3).

**Box 9.1**   Definitions of abuse categories.

*Physical injury*:   The actual or likely physical injury to a child, or failure to prevent physical injury (or suffering) to a child including deliberate poisoning, suffocation and Munchausen's syndrome by proxy.

*Sexual abuse*:   The actual or likely sexual exploitation of a child or adolescent. The child may be dependent and/or developmentally immature.

*Emotional abuse*:   The actual or likely adverse effect on the emotional and behavioural development of a child caused by persistent or severe emotional ill treatment or rejection.

*Neglect*:   The persistent or severe neglect of a child, or the failure to protect a child from exposure to any kind of danger, including cold and starvation, or extreme failure to carry out important aspects of care, resulting in the significant impairment of the child's health or development, including non-organic failure to thrive.

Adapted from *Working Together Under the Children Act 1989*[2].

**Box 9.2**   Physical abuse risk factors.

*Parental pressure*
- Premature baby/serious neonatal illness
- Handicapped child
- Failure to bond with baby/child
- Fretful/crying baby – difficult to console

*Environmental factors*
- Young, immature/inexperienced parents
- Social deprivation/drug and alcohol abuse
- Lack of good parenting models (persistent cycle of abuse)

**Box 9.3**   Clues to abuse.

- Delay in seeking medical help
- Clinical history vague or incompatible with injury
- Parent(s) preoccupied with self rather than concern for child
- Child appearance – frozen watchfulness occurs after repeated abuse
- Child may say something to raise suspicion

Hospitals will generally have a strict protocol as to the action to be taken when abuse is suspected and this will normally result in the referral of the patient to a consultant paediatrician who, in turn, will inform the necessary professional agencies.

The role of imaging in the examination of NAI is:

- To demonstrate and date clinically suspected fractures
- To demonstrate and date clinically occult fractures[8]

The skeletal survey is the main plain film examination undertaken when NAI is suspected but it is only appropriate for the examination of children under 2 years of age. Above this age, the use of alternative imaging strategies (MRI or scintigraphy) combined with confirmatory radiographic examination or selective radiography of clinically suspicious regions is more appropriate[8,9]. Imaging requests for NAI skeletal surveys should only be accepted from a paediatric consultant, preferably following discussion with a radiologist[10] as there is a large amount of inter-reliance between clinical and radiological evidence in the diagnosis of NAI[5].

The skeletal survey examination should be performed during normal working hours when the appropriate radiological expertise is available as this will prevent any unnecessary delay in the reporting of the examination or the recall of patients for additional projections. Each clinical department should have a skeletal survey protocol for use in cases of suspected physical abuse and, although the purpose of the skeletal survey is always to identify suggestive and occult skeletal injuries in order to confirm a suspected NAI diagnosis, the number and type of radiographic projections undertaken as part of the survey are not consistent between hospitals within the UK. This local variation may be as a result of radiologist preference, research evidence or traditional practice, but whatever the reason for the inclusion or exclusion of projections, it is important to ensure that the benefit to the patient from the examination outweighs the detriment/harm of exposure to radiation. In addition it is the radiographer's responsibility to ensure that the images produced are of optimum quality. A possible eight-projection skeletal survey is suggested in Box 9.4 but in addition to this, the following may also be considered necessary:

- Coned projections of fractures identified on the original survey or suspected metaphyseal/epiphyseal injuries
- Antero-posterior/postero-anterior skull projections (dependent on type and site of injury sustained)
- Dorsi-plantar hands and/or feet (if evidence of bruising/trauma present)

The correct diagnosis of NAI is imperative if further injury to the child is to be prevented and it is essential that all radiographs are of the highest quality as they may be submitted as evidence in a court of law. Anatomical markers, patient details and examination date/time should all be clearly marked on the film as well as the initials of the examining radiographer(s)[10]. The child should be accompanied to the imaging department by either the guardian(s), who should

**Box 9.4**  An example of an eight-projection skeletal survey.

Antero-posterior/postero-anterior chest (to image clavicles, ribs and scapulae)
Antero-posterior abdomen (to image spine and pelvis)
Antero-posterior both upper limbs (shoulder to metacarpals)
Antero-posterior both lower limbs (hip to tarsal bones)
Lateral thoracolumbar spine (to include spinous processes)
Lateral skull

be fully informed of the reasoning behind the imaging request, or a named nurse or social worker. It is important to remember that the role of the health care professional is not to 'judge' the patient or their families but to behave in a professional non-judgemental manner. Two radiographers (or radiographer plus assistant) should be present during the examination to act as witness to the proceedings[10,11] and it has been argued that within each imaging department a radiographer with specific responsibility for undertaking NAI skeletal surveys should be identified in order to optimise the radiographic image quality[11].

# Injury patterns

Accidental injury to non-ambulant infants is uncommon but does occasionally occur and therefore all cases must be reviewed in light of the social and historical evidence provided. For the majority of physically abused children there will be radiological evidence of skeletal injury[5] but cutaneous injuries, visible to the examining radiographer, may raise suspicions of physical abuse.

## *Cutaneous injury*

Bruises of varying ages are commonly found on young mobile children, particularly on the forearms and anterior aspects of the lower limbs, and it is important to distinguish accidental bruising from abuse. Bruising is present in approximately 90% of physical abuse cases[2] and the location, pattern, age and number of bruises can provide significant clues as to the likely cause of injury (Box 9.5). Finger tip bruises around the upper arms and chest wall suggest the child has been held tightly and therefore the possibility of the child being shaken must be considered[12]. Bruising around the pinna of the ear suggests 'boxing' or

**Box 9.5** Common bruising sites.

*Accidental bruising*
- Forehead
- Chin
- Spinous processes
- Iliac crests
- Forearms
- Shins

*Inflicted bruising*
- Ears
- Cheeks
- Neck
- Chest
- Abdomen
- Thighs
- Buttocks and genitalia

**Box 9.6**   Dating bruises[14].

| | |
|---|---|
| 1–2 days | Red, tender, swollen |
| 1–5 days | Blue/purple |
| 5–7 days | Green/yellow |
| 7–10 days | Yellow/brown |
| 1–4 weeks | Cleared |

'pinching' and tears to the frenulum of the upper lip are rarely accidental and usually result from a 'blow' to the mouth or 'forced' bottle feeding[13]. Other bruising may have an imprint of a weapon used (e.g. belt buckle or ring) or evidence of crescent-shaped nail markings and bite marks.

When considering bruising patterns and comparing the clinical history (time of injury) with the physical evidence, an awareness of the approximate age of bruises is important. However, the dating of bruises is not an exact science and variations occur between individual children (Box 9.6).

Burns and scalds, although uncommonly seen within the radiology department, are worth mentioning in this section for completeness. Neglected children are more prone to accidental burns (either from hot liquids or dry, hot surfaces) and careful consideration of the clinical history is essential before physical abuse is diagnosed. Accidental burns and scalds have characteristic drip, pour and splash patterns whereas hands, feet or buttocks that have been immersed in scalding water will have a 'glove' or 'stocking' pattern. Burns from hot objects may provide evidence of the shape of the object. However, cigarette burns, although apparently synonymous with abuse within many texts, are in reality uncommon injuries[12].

### Skeletal injury

#### Skull fracture

In children under 2 years of age, NAI is the foremost cause of serious head injury with up to 10% of physical abuse victims having evidence of a skull fracture[15] (Fig. 9.1). Damage to the brain as a result of physical abuse is not restricted to direct trauma to the skull but may also occur following forceful 'shaking' of an infant. Consideration of the clinical history and an understanding of trauma mechanisms are essential if an accurate diagnosis is to be made. A history of fall from a height of less than 1.25 m (4 feet) is rarely associated with a serious head injury[8] and therefore more sinister events need to be considered. No skull fracture pattern is pathognomonic of NAI but fractures of the parietal and occipital regions are more common than frontal bone fractures[2]. However, accidental skull fractures also typically present as simple linear fractures within the parietal region and therefore each case must be considered individually (Fig. 9.2).

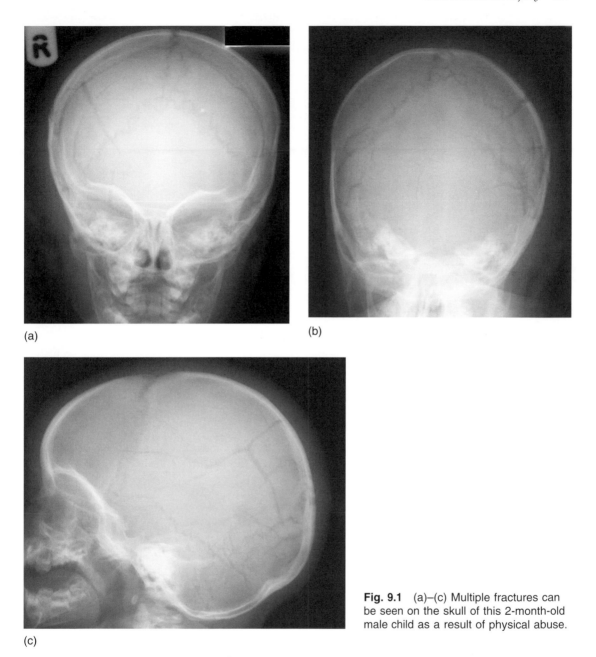

(a)

(b)

(c)

**Fig. 9.1**   (a)–(c) Multiple fractures can be seen on the skull of this 2-month-old male child as a result of physical abuse.

## Metaphyseal fracture

Metaphyseal fractures (where part or all of the rim of the metaphysis is separate) are often thought to be synonymous with NAI but are obvious only in the minority of cases[16]. They have been described as 'corner' or 'bucket handle' fractures but in reality they are identical and the different appearances are due to variations in the angle of the incident beam[5,16]. Metaphyseal fractures are often clinically occult and are not associated with symptoms of redness, pain, heat or

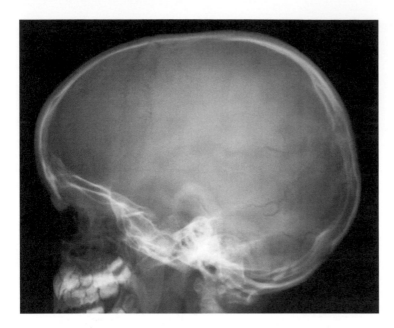

**Fig. 9.2**   A subtle linear fracture can be seen in the parietal region as a result of an accidental injury.

swelling. As a result, metaphyseal fractures are usually an incidental finding. The lower limbs are the commonest sites for metaphyseal fractures (knees and ankles) but any long bone metaphysis is susceptible as this is the area of most recent ossification and is the weakest part of the immature skeleton[17]. The dating of metaphyseal fractures is difficult as the healing process may occur without the formation of callus (Figs 9.3 and 9.4).

### Diaphyseal fractures

Diaphyseal fractures are the commonest non-accidental skeletal injury and are a highly suspicious indicator of abuse if found in non-ambulant infants[16]. A transverse fracture pattern presents more frequently than a spiral fracture but the latter is more suggestive of abuse as it results from a twisting force (Figs 9.5 and 9.6). The most commonly injured long bones are the humerus, femur and tibia; however, care must be taken not to confuse the fine spiral 'toddler' fracture (Chapter 7) with a physical abuse injury.

### Periosteal elevation

The periosteum is the outer sheath of bone and it consists of an inner osteogenic layer and an outer fibrous layer. Strong fibres bind the periosteum firmly to the epiphysis but these attachments are weaker along the disphyseal portion of the long bone and therefore periosteal elevation can occur following subperiosteal

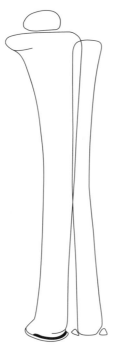

**Fig. 9.3** Distal metaphyseal 'corner' and 'bucket handle' fractures.

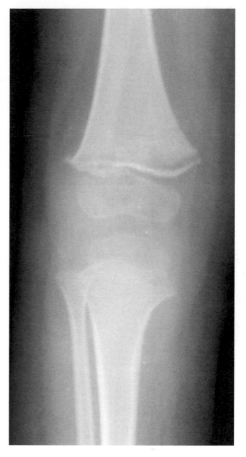

**Fig. 9.4** Metaphyseal fracture of the distal femur.

haemorrhage[16]. A variety of physical forces (e.g. twisting, grabbing, shaking) may produce a subperiosteal haemorrhage and periosteal elevation can be identified on radiographs at approximately 1 week post-trauma (Fig. 9.7). Periosteal elevation, although commonly seen on radiographs of physically abused children, is a non-specific condition and care should be taken when examining infants. It is thought that as a response to rapid growth, up to 40% of infants under 4 months of age will show radiographic evidence of periosteal reaction[5] but unlike a traumatic periosteal response, the appearances are symmetrical and do not extend to the metaphysis. Periosteal elevation is a clinically occult injury and healing is through gradual resorption and consolidation of new bone. Repeated trauma may result in multiple layers of periosteum and this may appear extensive.

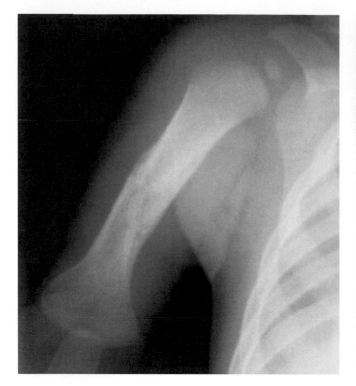

**Fig. 9.5**   Healing spiral fracture of the humerus.

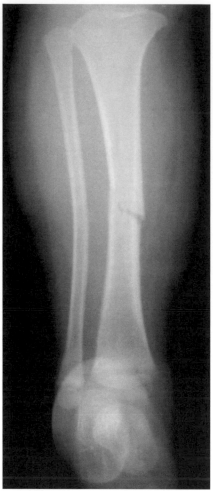

**Fig. 9.6**   A simple diaphyseal fracture thought to be caused accidentally until follow-up films demonstrated marked periosteal elevation (Fig. 9.7) suspicious of a twisting injury and non-accidental injury.

*Clavicle fractures*

The clavicle is one of the most commonly fractured bones in childhood but injuries as a result of abuse are seen in only 2–6% of patients. Accidental fractures tend to be located in the middle third of the clavicle (see Chapter 7) whereas fractures of the lateral end are uncommon accidental injuries and should raise suspicion of abuse (Fig. 9.8). The abusive mechanisms of clavicular fractures are uncertain. However, shaking and direct blunt trauma are possible causes[16].

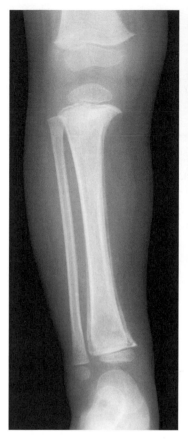

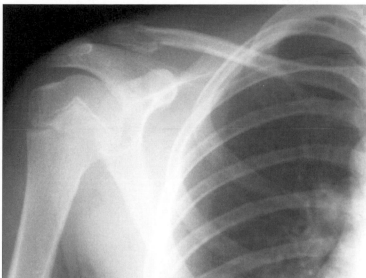

**Fig. 9.8** Fracture of the lateral portion of the clavicle.

**Fig. 9.7** Non-symmetrical periosteal elevation extending the metaphyseal regions of the tibia with associated proximal and distal metaphyseal fractures.

### Rib fractures

Accidental rib fractures, particularly those resulting from a compression injury of the thorax, are extremely uncommon in young children and therefore their presence is highly suspicious of abuse (Fig. 9.9). Rib fractures due to NAI are often multiple (commonly 6th–11th ribs[7]), bilateral and posterior[8]. They are thought to be present in up to 25% of cases although the majority are clinically occult[5]. Rib fractures may be difficult to diagnose radiographically when acute and therefore, if suspected, a repeat x-ray 7–12 days later (when fracture healing by callus formation can be identified) may be indicated. Alternatively, scintigraphy is sensitive to acute skeletal injuries.

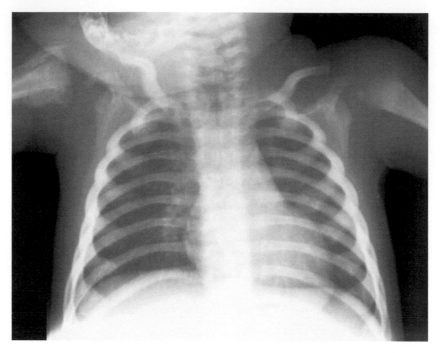

**Fig. 9.9** Healing anterior rib fractures are evident as well as marked raised periosteum around the proximal right humerus and associated acromion fracture.

### Vertebral fractures

Vertebral fractures due to NAI are rare but, should they occur, are usually located in the region of the thoracolumbar spine (Fig. 9.10). The mechanism of injury is commonly vigorous shaking of a young child resulting in hyperflexion of the spine. Radiographic evidence is typically height reduction at the anterior portion of the vertebral body with possible anterior endplate fractures and superior endplate extension. Avulsion of the spinous processes may also occur but as the tips of infant spinous processes are cartilaginous, this type of injury will not be apparent until calcification of the avulsed cartilage occurs[16].

### Digital fractures

Digital fractures (hands and feet) are uncommon in young children unless direct trauma has been experienced. Non-accidental injury to the hands and feet is usually the result of trampling, squeezing or hyperextension and, in the presence of a vague clinical history, digital fractures are suggestive of physical abuse.

## Summary

Non-accidental injury can present in many different forms and it has been the intention of this chapter to examine some of the more prevalent radiographic

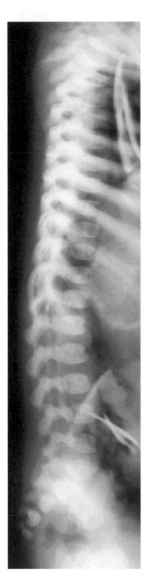

**Fig. 9.10** Lateral spine – post-mortem study. The child died as a victim of abuse. Note the typical appearances of paediatric vertebrae differ markedly from those of the adult patient.

appearances of NAI and emphasise the need for consistently high-quality radiographs. The summaries of injuries above are in no way intended to be exhaustive and Box 9.7 provides a list of injuries suggestive of NAI. However, it must be remembered that the presence of a suggestive injury is not proof of abuse and it is important to carefully consider the clinical and radiographic evidence together before confirming a diagnosis of physical abuse as other less sinister accidental and pathological conditions can have similar radiographic appearances.

**Box 9.7**  Skeletal fractures suggestive of non-accidental injury.

Metaphyseal fractures
Sternum and rib fractures
Vertebral fractures
Fracture of the scapula (particularly the acromion)
Fracture of the lateral end of the clavicle
Bilateral fractures
Multiple fractures of differing ages
Complex skull fractures (wider than 5 mm)
Digital fractures
Spiral fractures of the appendicular skeleton

# References

1. World Health Organisation (1997) *Child Abuse and Neglect: Fact Sheet N150* to be found at http://www.who.ch//
2. Department of Health (1991) *Working Together Under The Children Act 1989.* HMSO, London.
3. Warley, D. and Pettet, J. (1997) *Child Abuse: Recognition and Management.* Scutari Press, London.
4. Corby, B. (2000) *Child Abuse: Towards a Knowledge Base*, 2nd edn. Open University Press, Buckingham.
5. Carty, H., Shaw, D., Brunelle, F. and Kendall, B. (eds) (1994) *Imaging Children*, Volume 2. Churchill Livingstone, London.
6. NSPCC (1999) Published Figures of Children on Child Protection Registers.
7. Benson, M.K., Fixsen, J.A. and Macinol, M.F. (eds) (1994) *Children's Orthopaedics and Fractures.* Churchill Livingstone, London.
8. Rao, P. and Carty, H. (1999) Non-accidental injury: review of the radiology. *Clinical Radiology* **54**, 11–24.
9. Murray, I.P.C. and Ell, P.J. (eds) (1998) *Nuclear Medicine in Clinical Diagnosis and Treatment*, Volume 2, 2nd edn. Churchill Livingstone, London.
10. Cook, J.V., Pettet, A., Shah, K. *et al.* (1998) *Guidelines on Best Practice in the X-ray Imaging of Children: A Manual For All X-ray Departments.* Queen Mary's Hospital for Children, The St Helier NHS Trust, Carshalton, Surrey and The Radiological Protection Centre, St George's Healthcare NHS Trust, London.
11. Brown, A.M. and Henwood, S.M. (1997) Good practice for radiographers in non-accidental injury. *Radiography* **3**, 201–208.
12. Child Protection Committee, Bradford & Airedale NHS Trust (1996) *Signs and Symptoms of Child Abuse: A Guide for Staff.*
13. Blumenthal, I. (1994) *Child Abuse: A Handbook for Health Care Practitioners.* Edward Arnold, London.
14. Brown, G.J. (1997) *Principles and Practice of Children's Emergency Care.* MacLennon & Petty, London.
15. Meadow, R. (ed.) (1997) *ABC of Child Abuse*, 3rd edn. BMJ Publishing Group, London.
16. Kleinman, P.K. (1998) *Diagnostic Imaging of Child Abuse*, 2nd edn. Mosby, London.
17. Chew, F.S. (1996) *Skeletal Radiology: The Bare Bones.* Lippincott Williams & Wilkins, London.

# Index